CONTENTS

WA212

David H Hargreaves

Geoff W Southworth

Paula Stanley

Simon J Ward

ON-THE-JOB

TRAINING

FOR

PHYSICIANS

1 Wimpole Street, London WIM 8AE, UK
16 East 69th Street, New York, NY 10021, USA

British Library Cataloguing in Publication Data
A catalogue record for this book is available from the British Library
ISBN 1-85315-325-7

Cartoons by Graham Hagan, Charing, Kent
Design by Spot On Design, Leighton Buzzard, Bedfordshire
Phototypeset by Dobbie Typesetting Limited, Tavistock, Devon
Printed in Great Britain by Ebenezer Baylis, The Trinity Press, Worcester

FOREWORD

Pedagogy, like medicine, is an inexact pursuit. While science is about what we can know and theology is about what we may believe, education itself is neither truly a science nor a religion. Little of what we believe about education can be certain or immediately tested; like medicine it is subject to fashions and fads that can lead to radical and even hazardous changes of practice. Given the intrinsic uncertainties of medicine and pedagogy, how do medical educationists fit in?

Throughout history physicians have been differentiated clearly from other healers by the expectations placed upon them; they were privileged by their education and unique traditions of practice so that even the early universities provided for their vocation. For thousands of years doctors have educated doctors in the art and emerging science of medicine. They have served the public well and no-one would seriously suggest that a societal experiment with a withdrawal of medical practitioners from a society as a whole should be undertaken.

Well-doctored societies only have to examine those where a rigorous university training in medicine is not available to shrink from the experiment but another uncontrolled trial is already well under way in England and Wales; the rapid introduction of the so-called Calman reforms in specialist training have questioned the long-practised apprenticeship concept that has been allied to responsible service work in the postgraduate training. A new career structure has been introduced with a marked reduction of the periods of professional training required. Thus training will be accomplished for specialist accreditation at the consultant level within a greatly-reduced period.

These changes, introduced without pilot work or fair trial, pose difficulties for postgraduate medical trainees and the senior staff who are obliged to teach them. Moreover, the changes have occurred at a time of profound change in all the professions; in the funding of education; in the management of the health service; in university administration and in society generally. They have been brought in at a time of rapid social transformation; they were initiated by a doctrinaire (and now deposed) administration wishing to ingratiate itself with the common man.

The arguments are familiar and already well-rehearsed; these changes are anathema to many doctors and senior staff — those who have grown up in a system that

v

espoused the commitment of the universities and the National Health Service to medical education on a knock-to-knock basis over half a century. This guide is to be welcomed, it is based on a genuine and bold desire by David Hargreaves, Geoff Southworth, Paula Stanley and Simon Ward to examine clinical vocational training by consultants and other staff in several specialties and in different hospitals throughout East Anglia during the time the reforms were being introduced. The team meticulously investigated teaching practice conducted by clinical staff at all hours. They not only took soundings, they developed ideas, tested them with volunteers, returned to describe their experiences and responses and, by consensus, have distilled key ideas and practice as well as techniques of training used for the education of medical postgraduates.

The authors are active in education research as applied to medicine. They are aware of the pitfalls of a quasi-objective approach to pedagogy, of the remorseless criticism of hard-working senior doctors and the sheer complexity of medical practice. They understand the concept of the mentor and the hero or heroine character and the need for feedback and encouragement in clinical skills. They have analysed as simply as possible aspects of vocational training and how knowledge of the whole patient can be integrated in the sight of the patient by a thoughtful teacher.

This then is an inspired and accessible guide that should enable teacher and trainee to make the best use of their limited (and mutually precious) time together. For the student, the integration of knowledge means that what is important is what survives when what is learned has been forgotten. For the teacher the inducement must be the glimpse of immortality hinted at by Henry Adams: *A teacher affects eternity; he can never tell where his influence stops*. I commend this guide to you.

Timothy M Cox
Professor of Medicine, Cambridge

PREFACE

Reforms in specialist training in the United Kingdom have challenged physicians in their thinking about postgraduate training. While instruction of medical students has been by rote for generations with the teacher delivering accepted wisdom to a forbearing audience, the last 30 years have seen a challenge to this concept with the introduction of problem-based learning and small group teaching.

Clinical training for both students and postgraduates has long accepted these principles, especially in bedside teaching and clinics, through observation, instruction and supervised practice. The challenge presented by the new specialist training for physicians is to make learning of clinical medicine more effective and more efficient. This is what the team from the University of Cambridge has set out to do, through observing and working with medical teachers and postgraduate trainees in wards and clinics and theatres in a number of associated hospitals.

On-the-job training epitomises the clinical approach in its most constructive form; its acceptance will be a significant contribution to success of specialist training for physicians and will find endorsement by all willing to accept the challenge of the new system. This guide will help to carry the process forward and I offer my congratulations to David Hargreaves and the team.

John SG Biggs
Postgraduate Dean
January 1997

INTRODUCTION

The challenge

Following the Calman reforms and the New Deal, the training time between appointment as a Senior House Officer (SHO), through the Specialist Registrar grade, to achieving the status of a specialist and taking up a consultancy is to be much reduced—a shorter working week over fewer years. So the quality and quantity of training needs to be improved. This Guide is designed to meet the changing needs and demands for training that now impinge on SHOs, Specialist Registrars and Consultants in medical specialities.

What is to be done?

> We need to look again at how doctors learn and how teaching methods can be improved in order that time spent in education can be used efficiently. Supervision and feedback are crucial . . . The integration of theoretical teaching with practical work, progressive assessment and feedback to teachers and trainees are essential.
> Sir Kenneth Calman, Chief Medical Officer, 1993[1]

Is there a problem?

Concern about the quality of training has a long history.

> In only one respect has there been a decided lack of progress in the domain of medicine, that is in the time it takes to become a qualified practitioner. In the good old days a man was turned out thoroughly equipped after putting in two winter sessions at a college and spending his summers in running logs for a sawmill. Nowadays it takes anywhere from five to eight years to become a doctor. It seems odd that a man should study eight years now to learn what he used to acquire in eight months.
> Stephen Leacock, economist and humorist, 1910

> No progress has as yet been made towards formulating the concept of the clinician as teacher. It is still supposed that because a man is an accomplished physician he is an excellent teacher. Clinical teaching in London remains an incident in the life of a busy Consultant.
> Abraham Flexner, reformer of medical education, 1910

It is widely recognised that the outcomes of British postgraduate medical training are good. The degree of junior doctors' satisfaction with training in more recent times is, however, variable. Several surveys indicate that many trainees are critical of some of the ways in which they are trained.

EVALUATIONS OF POSTGRADUATE TRAINING

Formally defined teaching rounds for PGME are uncommon . . . Most Consultant PGME teaching appears to be provided in general ward rounds (business rounds). The teaching element is rarely defined . . . There is relatively little formal teaching in outpatients . . . For the majority of trainees, educational opportunities within outpatients were *ad hoc* . . . The most common criticism levelled by trainees was that they did not have the opportunity to examine, treat and learn about complex cases . . . [2]

Most trainees want more and better training. Under ten per cent believe training is given a high priority by their seniors. Almost half the SHOs believe more time could and should be given to their training, though the pressure of clinical work-loads is recognised. Some believe more use could be made of Registrars in the training of SHOs and that their existing contribution could be better recognised. Many trainees receive little feedback on progress in training. The feedback provided tends to be sparse, haphazard, implicit and indirect.[3]

The responses obtained to the questionnaire indicate the large extent to which SHOs are in a grade which includes training only in name. The finding is largely consistent across all survey specialties and hospital types . . . This paper shows that there is very little systematic teaching, few available good teachers and that learning is very much an *ad hoc* process . . . Just over half the SHOs cited Registrars or Senior Registrars as providing some teaching . . . That only about half of SHOs cite Consultants as providing most of their teaching is dramatic and a figure for concern . . . SHOs opted for Senior Registrars and Registrars as their preferred teachers rather than Consultants.[4]

Towards a solution of the problem

General professional training of 2 to 3 years in the SHO grade with acquisition of the MRCP (UK) leads to the specialist registrar grade in about 5 years and the Certificate of Completion of Specialist Training (CCST). Improvement in the quality of formal training is taking place at all levels but this raises the issue of how well formal training is articulated with on-the-job training. Improvements are needed in both, together with better linking, if training as a whole is to become more coherent and more effective.

Junior doctors see on-the-job training—where training is combined with, and runs alongside, service delivery—as important, and will doubtless continue to do so. Yet little has been written on how this is best done. The Guide explains how trainers and trainees can improve on-the-job training for physicians.

THE NEW TRAINING

Because the training period will be shorter, and educational standards must be maintained, the training element in all training grade posts must be strengthened. Service work done must complement training rather than interfere with it.[5]

An aspect that will be new to many is the introduction of training agreements between the trainee, postgraduate dean, and the hospital trust(s) where training is to take place . . . Key elements [include] the structure and aims of the teaching programme and the standards of achievement expected of the trainee; an explanation of the methods and frequency of assessment; a commitment by Consultants to regular in-service tuition; and protected time for trainees to study and be trained. There will also be a commitment from the trainee to take an active part in the training.[6]

Our training, it would be fair to say, is in a state of flux. There's always been the 'learn by what you do' approach, but with the Calman changes we have to focus on what we Consultants are doing for the trainees and what they're getting out of it. It's no longer sufficient for us to assume that the training happens.[7]

I never feel that my knowledge is right, I don't feel that the whole thing comes together unless there's a patient involved. For the best way to learn medicine is almost the traditional way—round the patient. The more you do away from the patient, separately in the lecture theatre, the less you can get the whole thing together in your mind. The balance has to be skewed towards being with patients, on the ward and in clinic. The best way is not to take trainees out and give them more lectures. That's easier for the bosses to monitor, but I'm not convinced that it's the best way of doing it. You mustn't take people away from the working environment where they learn.[8]

The Guide:

- helps trainers (Consultants, Specialist Registrars) to train more effectively
- helps Consultants and Specialist Registrars to work as partners in training SHOs
- helps trainees (Specialist Registrars, SHOs) to get the best out of training.

Teaching can also help one to learn. When one teaches, one tests out and refines the quality and depth of one's own knowledge, skill and understanding. The Guide helps Specialist Registrars to teach and to learn through teaching.

The Guide is grounded in a research and development project, sponsored by the Postgraduate Dean and funded by the Anglia Postgraduate Medical and Dental Education Committee. The project sought to identify good practice in different specialties in different hospitals. Doctors who volunteered to take part in the project are among those committed to improving training. We do not claim they are typical, but the settings and circumstances in which they work are to be found everywhere. Ideas developed during the project were tested out by volunteers. Wherever possible trainers and trainees speak in their own words to describe their experiences and their responses to training, both old and new. Naturally, they remain anonymous.

REFERENCES

1 Calman KC. Medical education: a look into the future. *Postgrad Med Education J* 1993; **69**: (supplement 2) S3–S5.
2 Barker A, Scotland AD, Challah S, Gainey B, Bailey IA. A comparative study of postgraduate medical eduction in North East Thames Region. *Postgrad Med J* 1994; **70**: 722–7.
3 Booth M, Bradley H, Hargreaves DH, Southworth G. Unpublished survey of junior doctors, 1994.
4 Grant J, Marsden P, King RC. Senior house officers and their training. *BMJ* 1989; **299**: 1263–8.
5 Committee of Postgraduate Medical Deans and UK Conference of Postgraduate Deans. *SHO training: tackling the issues, raising the standards*, 1995.
6 Biggs J. New arrangement for specialist training in Britain: guidance notes for implementing the specialist registrar grade. *BMJ* 1995; **311**: 1242–3.
7 Quotation from transcript of interview with Consultant Physician, 1996.
8 Quotation from transcript of interview with Trainee, 1996.

HOW TO USE THE GUIDE

> *There is a profound gap between applicable and actionable knowledge. The former tells you what is relevant; the latter tells you how to implement it in the world of everyday practice.*
>
> Chris Argyris and Donald Schön, educationists, 1974

It is easy, on the basis of sound educational principles, to offer advice on how to improve the training of doctors in hospitals—e.g. trainers should give trainees more feedback. This is just applicable knowledge, which trainers may know and understand but with no noticeable impact on their training practices.

The Guide aims at actionable knowledge, which explains precisely how to implement the advice in the everyday life of a hospital.

The Guide is divided into four Parts.

Part One and Part Four deal with the **key ideas**—on-the-job training, osmosis and coaching, the meaning of progression, education and training.

Part Two describes the basic **techniques** of training—asking questions, explaining, giving feedback.

Part Three focuses on the **settings** where you put these training techniques into action—clinics, wards and on-take.

Select Sections according to your interest rather than reading from cover to cover.

How TRAINERS might use the Guide

The ideal way to use this Guide is when all the Consultants in a department:

- commit themselves to making training a high priority and to improving everybody's skills at both learning and teaching
- decide that they will use the Guide to help to change training practices
- involve the whole department, Consultants, Specialist Registrars and SHOs and all other professional staff with the aim of creating a training culture
- treat Specialist Registrars both as trainees and, under the supervision of the Consultants, as contributors to the training of SHOs.

If the whole team shares the same goal, success is achieved more quickly.

Skim read Parts One and Four, then focus on those Sections in Parts Two and Three which you believe will be most important for you. Section 10 in Part Three discusses written training plans which may require agreement among all the trainers. Some parts of the Guide will simply reflect what you already do. Others will give you ideas for developing those aspects of training you would like to improve.

Teaching in on-the-job training (OJT), like any other skill in medicine, takes time and practice to learn. You can no more read advice on how to train effectively and then immediately put it into successful practice than you can read about a procedure and then carry it out easily and with total success. Skill in teaching is best acquired step by step. So focus on, and master, one aspect at a time.

Some Sections could be used, in whole or part, for a departmental discussion, in protected time for formal training, to discuss approaches to, and strategies for, OJT. Talking through the members' feelings and ideas about OJT is a good way of creating interest in improving its quality. All the Sections in Parts Two and Three can be used in this way. Sections 5 and 9 in Part Two should provoke stimulating debate.

How TRAINEES might use the Guide

As a junior doctor, you will use the Guide mainly to help you

- make the most of the on-the-job training offered to you
- learn how to identify more opportunities for learning within the daily routines of service delivery
- exploit those opportunities more fully by learning how to elicit better training from all those with whom you are working.

Start by skim reading Sections 2 and 4 in Part One and then move to Section 5 in Part Two on taking control of your learning. You will then probably pick out those Sections in Part Two (techniques) and Part Three (settings) that are of interest and relevance to you. You will find it useful to read Section 10 in Part Three, whether or not you have an official training plan, since some of the ideas there can help you plan your on-the-job learning for yourself.

Learning from OJT, like any other skill in medicine, takes time and practice. You can no more read advice on getting the best out of training and then immediately put it into successful practice than you can read about a procedure and then carry it out easily and with total success. Skill in learning is best acquired step by step. So focus on, and master, one aspect at a time.

Choose **one** Section on which to work for a time. When you have made progress in that area, turn to another topic. It is impractical to work on all Sections at once.

How 'TRAIN THE TRAINER' COURSE LEADERS might use the Guide

Such courses will increasingly be concerned with training trainers to be more effective in OJT as well as in formal training sessions. The Guide may be used:

- as a complement to work on various kinds of formal and off-the-job training
- as a resource for clarifying the nature of OJT and its theoretical and conceptual infrastructure (Parts One and Four)
- as a text or resource book for training sessions on OJT
- as the basis for designing activities and exercises on either the techniques of OJT or the application of the techniques in action settings.

Each Section ends with a set of Action Points, which may be treated as an *aide-mémoire*, copied onto cards or into a filofax and be carried in a white coat pocket.

I   TRAINING AS APPRENTICESHIP — OSMOSIS OR COACHING?

> *In postgraduate medical education, 'apprenticeship' is the accepted dominant model of training — defined as learning by doing under the supervision of an experienced practitioner . . . This model, if unanalysed, perpetuates the unhelpful confusion between training and service, to the extent that providing the service may become identified with receiving training . . . But learning by doing, in the absence of a teacher to provide guidance and feedback, has the inherent potential of learning the wrong thing in the wrong way . . .*
>
> J Grant, P Marsden and RC King, medical educators, 1989
>
> *The term on-the-job training is one I abhor, because it generally implies that people will pick things up as they go along. We think, as we do in many cases of apprentice- ships, that putting a young person with someone experienced will automatically transfer knowledge and theory. The developmental responsibility of the coach- manager is much broader than that.*
>
> Sir John Harvey-Jones, industrialist, 1994
>
> *How are skills learned? By experience. How, then, are they best taught? By coaching.*
>
> Theodore Sizer, educationist, 1984

THIS SECTION
- **explains the difference between the two major models of apprenticeship**
- **describes the strengths of apprenticeship by coaching**

In talking about training, doctors commonly use two words — 'osmosis' and 'apprenticeship'.

Osmosis refers to the vague processes by which, during the daily round of service delivery, a trainee somehow 'picks up' relevant knowledge, skills and under- standing.

It is an unplanned and unsystematic yet pervasive feature of professional learning. Much is acquired simply by watching and listening to colleagues as well as directly through 'hands-on' experience. Osmosis includes modelling by the trainer and incidental learning, where a trainee incidentally gains some knowledge or skill when primarily intending to reach some other goal. There is also coincidental learning when the trainee happens to be around as the Consultant encounters a rare condition.

I

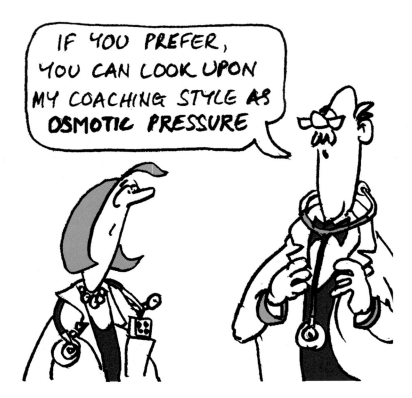

An apprenticeship model of training does not exclude elements of osmosis — learning simply by being around the trainer or imitating the trainer after a period of close observation. But true apprenticeship — a model of training widely adopted in a variety of professions and trades in the past — extends far beyond osmosis, for there is planned, systematic and deliberate teaching. 'Sitting next to Nellie' — the phrase often used to describe the industrial version of the osmotic apprenticeship — becomes a more effective form of training when she takes her responsibilities seriously and willingly assumes an active role in shaping the apprentice's learning.

The effective 'master' traditionally coached the apprentice by:

- demonstrating knowledge and skill
- being a role model in how to relate to colleagues and clients
- providing a lot of hands-on experience
- guiding the apprentice through regular practice
- setting clear objectives and targets to support the apprentice's learning
- supervising progression through the steps that lead to mastery
- having sufficient self-restraint to resist doing the job for the apprentice

2

- seeing the apprentice as a help to his/her own work, not as a hindrance to it
- accepting that a bright apprentice is a person the master can learn with and from.

If the trainer offers structured training that is intentional, planned, monitored and followed up, then it is the apprenticeship-by-coaching model. If it is not, then it is the unstructured, and educationally much inferior, apprenticeship-by-osmosis model, where the teaching and learning is unplanned, unsystematic and unsupported.

THE LIMITS OF APPRENTICESHIP-BY-OSMOSIS

Training is more informal [than in the US], it's much more an apprenticeship in the UK. We leave a lot more to the trainees' initiative and let them choose what they learn. I think our training system encourages that. It isn't spoon-feeding.

Consultant

We all know that we've learnt what we do by apprenticeship. We'd be saying we were inadequate in our jobs if we said that was wrong. We're not going to say that because we seem to get our patients through fairly well, so we feel that the way we were trained is adequate.

Consultant

Some Consultants are distant and arrogant because they spent so long being treated badly by the system that when they make the grade, they treat their juniors badly— you know, the argument that the system produced me so it can't be all that bad. They think that the teaching we get is purely by exposure and that that's adequate.

Trainee

There is no on-the-job training. You just pick it up, just like an apprentice.

Trainee

3

APPRENTICESHIP-BY-COACHING:
the views of some trainers

I'm quite sure that I learnt most from the other more senior trainees I was with, Regis-
trars and Senior Registrars, and it was a very good relationship; I learnt by feeling that
I knew them well enough to sit down and chat. That is certainly the way that I learnt, in
a very informal way. An informal process and unstructured to that degree fails when
there is too much work to do or too little time.

Consultant

I don't think teaching is all one-way. You learn yourself all the time by teaching. Some-
times a trainee asks you a simple question which goes right to the heart of something,
which you probably haven't thought about for a while and then you realise that, yes, it's
a good question and you begin to wonder 'Did I ever really understand it myself?'

Consultant

I don't know what happens to people when they become Consultants. They forget what
they went through. When I become one, I won't leave my juniors like that. I'll try to give
them the best on-the-job training I can because I feel very strongly about the way I've
had to struggle.

Registrar

Trainers who perpetuate apprenticeship-by-osmosis on the grounds that if it was good enough for them it should be good enough for their trainees, ignore the fact that the knowledge, skills and techniques which trainees now have to acquire are greater than in the past and have to be acquired during a much shorter training. Some trainers have reacted critically towards their own training under the apprenticeship-by-osmosis model and have adopted a model in which the trainer is a coach. Other trainers have been trained under an apprenticeship-by-coaching model and want to continue with the approach to training they found valuable. They are convinced it is the way forward.

THE MERITS OF APPRENTICESHIP-BY-COACHING
a psychological viewpoint

It is held by psychologists that there is an important space between what a learner is able to do independently and what he or she might do with the active support of, or in collaboration with, a more experienced person. How the coach 'tells' or 'explains' or 'questions' the trainee can effect the closing of that space. Good teaching can serve as a kind of scaffolding around the skill or knowledge to be acquired, so that with its help, the trainee moves beyond what he or she could do alone. Through the teaching techniques adopted and the way they are put into practice, the coach provides scaffolding for the skills and knowledge that are, without help, just out of the apprentice's reach but, with help, within it.

Trainees, like all learners, experience the difficulty of applying what they know in an academic or intellectual sense. On-the-job training is rich in possibilities for teaching by scaffolding for three reasons:

- It is in OJT that a trainer detects and documents that the trainee has only partially mastered a skill and needs help.

- It is in OJT that the trainer can then provide the scaffolding or active help by which the trainee is able to demonstrate the skill that could not have been done alone.

- It is in OJT that the trainer can subsequently monitor the trainee's exercise of the skill and be satisfied that it is indeed mastered.

2 UNDERSTANDING ON-THE-JOB TRAINING

> *Until proper educational analysis of the contribution of service work to training is done, the enforced dominant model — of service being training — will persist.*
>
> J Grant, P Marsden and RC King, medical educators, 1989
>
> *All Consultants have a part to play: the role of the majority will be to facilitate apprenticeship learning through routine service work . . . Informal and opportunistic learning should be valued highly as an important component of the overall educational package available to doctors in training . . . It should be developed and supported to increase its educational effectiveness.*
>
> The Report of SCOPME, 1994
> (The Standing Committee on Postgraduate Medical Education)

THIS SECTION
- **describes the types of training**
- **explains why OJT needs to be:**
  - **planned rather than opportunistic**
  - **fusional rather than intrusive**
  - **cyclical rather than fragmented**
  - **an investment rather than a duty**

The types of training are:
- 'off-the-job' or formal training
- 'on-the-job' training (OJT), which is either informal or semi-formal.

Formal, off-the-job training occurs when teaching and learning are the only activities being intentionally undertaken and neither is directly related to any current or ongoing service delivery or patient under treatment. Lectures, seminars and courses are obvious examples. Formal training usually occurs in a dedicated place e.g. a seminar room.

OJT — informal training — takes place with a real case during service, usually with the patient present. The main settings for OJT are wards, clinics and on-take.

OJT — semi-formal training — is triggered by real cases during service but diverges from the case at hand into broader issues. Semi-formal training occurs, for instance, on a teaching ward round when the trainer discusses issues of diagnosis or

6

management which link to but are not directly related to the patient before them. In some semi-formal situations — a meeting prior to the ward round, a case presentation session or a meeting to study patients' X-rays — the patients are not present.

Semi-formal situations are often seen by trainees as especially rich in opportunities for teaching and learning, mainly because the issues are seen as relevant to their practice and the lack of immediate pressure from the demands of service delivery provides the 'space' for discussion. A common example is when a trainee in clinic goes to get advice on how to manage a patient and then through that short conversation gets some teaching as well as a solution to a service problem.

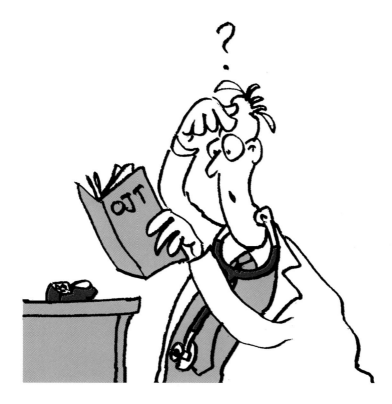

7

The features of effective on-the-job training

Apprenticeship-by-coaching involves a distinctive philosophy and set of practices that can be explained in terms of the following distinctions. That is, OJT is:

- planned rather than just opportunistic
- fusional rather than intrusive
- cyclical rather than fragmented
- an investment rather than a duty.

Planned *versus* opportunistic OJT

Much OJT has an opportunistic character. The trainer takes the line that training is contingent on the cases that turn up when the trainee is around to be taught, and when there is sufficient time to engage in the teaching. Since, the argument runs, both variables are difficult to predict or control, trainee and trainer are destined to take a 'wait and see' line and make the most of any opportunities that arise.

From the perspective of apprenticeship-by-coaching, opportunistic OJT has several faults:

- it is a re-active rather than a pro-active philosophy, inducing in both trainer and trainee a fatalism that they are at the mercy of events rather than the masters of them
- it under-estimates the degree to which some aspects of both training and service delivery are predictable and open to control through planning
- it discourages both trainer and trainee from scanning service delivery for opportunities for OJT and then exploiting them in the interests of the trainee.

Planned OJT does not deny that OJT is indeed subject to the severe constraints of service pressures and the chance of what turns up in the case-load, but sees these as constraints upon training rather than as insurmountable barriers to it. OJT is not open to the kind of planning appropriate to formal training — deciding beforehand exactly what will be taught at what point in what sequence. OJT is, however, open to planning that is more flexible and readily adaptable in the light of experience and changing circumstances.

How to plan training is the subject of Section 10, p. 75.

Fusional *versus* intrusive OJT

Trainers and trainees often contrast training with service — one is doing either the one or the other. This is natural enough for we put a mental frame around our actions in the light of our intentions. If we intend to teach, our action is framed as 'training': if we intend to treat patients, our action is framed as 'service'.

Sometimes training interrupts service delivery because the trainer, in order to teach, stops the service to start teaching (e.g. explains, or asks the trainee some questions, or demonstrates a skill to the trainee) and so takes longer to complete the service. As trainers rightly see such training as intrusive of service, they say there is insufficient time for training. On-the-job training is fine, the argument goes, but the job takes longer than it would otherwise do and that cannot be afforded.

OJT does not, however, always have to be intrusive. A second and far more significant form, which we might call fusional OJT, is when the OJT is fused with service, that is, the training is integrated, and takes place simultaneously, with service delivery. Intentions fuse, so frames fuse too. One is indeed doing two things at once.

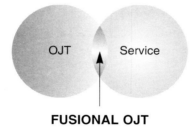

FUSIONAL OJT

OJT can mean learning then doing: fusional OJT means learning whilst doing. In fusional OJT the job often takes no more time than if no training were taking place. There are two types of fusional OJT:

- **Single track**, as when the trainer is carrying out a procedure and simultaneously provides a running commentary to explain that procedure to the trainee; and
- **Double track**, as when the trainer carries out a procedure and simultaneously talks to the trainee about something relevant to the case, but not about the procedure that the trainer is doing.

EXAMPLES OF FUSIONAL OJT

- the trainer asks the trainee a question without stopping the physical examination of the patient

- during a ward round the trainer explains to the patient and the trainees present the nature of the treatment that has been selected

- the trainee who is seeking advice from the trainer in clinic is asked to examine the patient in a way that allows the trainee to learn but does not require the trainer to make a separate or independent examination.

Fusional OJT is an efficient and effective form of OJT, but producing it in quantity and with quality is a highly skilled activity. There are two major components:

The first is the psychological change of abandoning the view that one can handle only one frame at a time — either teaching or service delivery. The two frames are combined in fusional OJT. The coach moves from thinking or saying 'There just isn't enough time for teaching' to 'What opportunities are there in the next hour for any fusional OJT?' Every piece of service delivery in which coach and trainee are co-present contains potential for fusional OJT.

The second component is the practical skill of learning how to insert the maximal amount of fusional OJT into service and reduce intrusive OJT to a minimum.

Service is richer in opportunities for training than most trainers and trainees realise. Both coach and trainee have to learn how to scan the service in which they are jointly engaged, in order to recognise the opportunities and then exploit them to the full.

Cyclical *versus* fragmented OJT

Ideally OJT has the structure of a coaching cycle with three phases.

PHASES OF A COACHING CYCLE

- a **planning phase** where coach and trainee decide the aspect of training on which to focus

- a **service delivery phase** into which OJT is fused or blended

- a **follow-up phase** where coach and trainee review the quality of trainee performance and any training provided and decide what to do in the next training cycle.

In practice, coaching cycles rarely take this ideal, cyclical form, since both the planning and follow-up phases are left out. The structure of OJT is often highly fragmented, and sometimes for good reason. Since some OJT is necessarily opportunistic, a formal planning phase may not be possible. In the same way, OJT often slides back into service delivery and there is neither the time nor the opportunity for any follow-up discussion — and sometimes no appropriate private place in which to conduct it.

OJT as an investment *versus* training as a duty — training pays!

The best planning is guided by a conception of training as an investment:

- a short-term investment — faster and better service delivery
- a long-term investment — a better Consultant in due course.

Training treated as a duty is a natural partner of OJT conceived as necessarily intrusive and opportunistic. But training can and should be seen also as an investment, not merely in the self-evident sense of contributing to the development of the trainee, but also in the less obvious sense of making a highly effective contribution to current service delivery, including the work-load of the trainer.

In medicine there are cases in clinics and aspects of patient care on the ward, that are appropriately handed over to trainees. If the acquisition of some of the relevant knowledge and skill by trainees occurs very soon after their arrival in the firm or

11

department, this frees the trainer to get on with those aspects of service delivery that are too important or difficult to be delegated.

The element of investment is this: ensuring that trainees acquire some relevant knowledge and skills at a very early stage does require time and effort from the trainer, both to teach the relevant knowledge and skill and then to provide the close supervision to check that trainees can carry out the relevant clinical tasks effectively. But the trainer's time saved in subsequent weeks or months more than compensates for the initial outlay of trainer time. Moreover, trainees see that their training is being made a priority and that they are making speedy progress at an early stage. As a result their morale and confidence rise rapidly, which makes a more committed and competent trainee. Therefore the investment in training pays off in several ways.

For training to be such a sound investment it has to be planned by the coach with great care. OJT occurs in a range of settings — wards, clinics and on-take — and a sound plan takes account of what can best be learned in one particular setting.

> You've got investment as far as the hospital's concerned. If you are trained, you are able to perform your job more efficiently at an earlier stage, rather than basically trying to learn it as you go along. You become an effective doctor and you can be left unsupervised at an earlier stage.
>
> Trainee

> One of the advantages of having trainees is that you can do other things. Let's be blunt about it. This idea that everything will be done by the Consultant and the junior will only learn is wrong-headed. Juniors will always have to do some work, in part because the system cannot cope without them working too and in part, if they watch they can't really develop the practical skills. There comes a point where they have to do things and the doing is part of the service. And whilst I'm watching or supervising whilst they're getting on with it, I can be doing something else at the same time. That's economics.
>
> Trainer

> When I was a houseman, I had two house jobs, one in which I was taught fairly frequently, whether it be bedside or formally, and I got a lot out of that job. And the other job, you had to pick it up as you went along without much help and training, and so I got very little out of that job. It's easy to know which I'm more competent in.
>
> Trainee

Learning without coaching

The coach helps the trainee to learn, but this does not always mean that the coach must be engaged in teaching. It means, rather, that the coach ensures that the trainee is placed in conditions where learning can take place. On-the-job learning by a trainee often occurs in conditions where the trainer is not even present.

Trainees must be in a position to profit from their own experience. Learning to recognise clinical conditions in patients and to make judgements about them, along continua such as normal/abnormal, common/rare, trivial/serious or superficial/extensive, requires exposure to many actual examples as well as text-book knowledge. Interpersonal skills, e.g. the appropriate ways in which to relate to nursing and paramedical staff, or breaking bad news to patients or relatives, are learned through experience as well as observation of role models.

Coaches can help trainees to see the importance of learning through experience if they point out what can be learned in this way and in which settings. Work on wards and clinics can seem unduly boring to trainees if they ignore the fact that seeing common cases with high frequency provides the essential background for recognising important variations of the condition and, allows the mental processes underlying such recognition to move from being slow and analytical to becoming faster and more intuitive. Learning-on-the-job in the absence of explicit teaching is an important but under-estimated part of OJT.

13

3 THE PARTNERSHIPS IN COACHING

> The [trainee] cannot be taught what he needs to know but he can be coached.
>
> Donald Schön, educationist, 1987
>
> In my training you had to be very motivated to get the most out of your training. You had to be very rigorous in making sure that you got time for your learning and didn't allow yourself to be side-tracked into doing entirely service commitment. I really think now that the culture is changing and there's more recognition that there's a minimum amount of time all juniors must have for their training. I think now it's much more a joint responsibility of the trainer and trainee.
>
> Consultant, 1996

THIS SECTION OUTLINES

- **the partnership created between coach and trainee**
- **the partnership between Consultant and Specialist Registrar as trainers**
- **the responsibilities and rewards of being a coach and a trainee**

In apprenticeship-by-osmosis, the trainer leaves most of the responsibility for learning with the trainee. In apprenticeship-by-coaching, the trainer and trainee accept a range of responsibilities but in turn receive significant rewards.

The **responsibilities of the coach** are to:

- show a real commitment to training
- take the lead with trainees in making a plan for training and to take part in the plan's implementation
- support trainees through encouragement and through boosting their self-confidence
- provide opportunities for learning that are appropriate to the trainee's needs
- take an active role in training by using a range of teaching methods
- give feedback, both positive and negative
- help the trainee to assess the rate and extent of progress in learning
- evaluate whether what was planned has in fact been achieved.

Unless these are evident, you cannot expect your trainees to be very committed either to the training or to the job itself. On-the-job training means that when the training is good the job also is done better.

The trainer needs to be aware of, and sensitive to, each trainee's career intention and current status in relation to college examinations, for such factors affect trainees' learning needs at any one time. The variations include:

- one who wishes to pursue the trainer's specialty
- one who wants to pursue another medical specialty
- one who wants to be a GP
- one who remains as yet undecided.

The physician trainer has a distinct advantage over the surgeon in providing an appropriate training for the GP trainee registrars.

> The emphasis of a specialist physician is to reach a very clear diagnosis and to have a very clear plan of management, starting with the easier things and then moving to the more complex. There's no fundamental difference between us and GPs; it's just a matter of detail really; we all remain physicians.
>
> Consultant Physician
>
> One of the important things you do for trainees is impart the specialist's way of thinking into their heads. Take the difference between the way a GP and a surgeon thinks about a patient. The GP thinks about the signs and symptoms, how bad the condition is, what the first line of treatment is, whether referral will be necessary if things don't improve and so on. Whereas what the surgeon thinks about centres around the question: do I need to operate or not? And what I look for is a prognostic reason for operating or a symptomatic reason for operating. If both are present the decision is easier. What you are looking for is an indication to operate or an absence of an indication to operate. This is at the heart of the process of decision making for a surgeon. But that is not the way a GP would look at the same condition. Trainees can get lost in a sea of information, or can give undue weight to some information or ignore some information which is relevant. There is a definite way of thinking for a specialist of every sort and you have to try to impart that way of thinking to your trainees.
>
> Consultant Surgeon

Every trainee has a right to have his/her distinctive position respected by the trainer.

The **rewards for the coach** are:

- a trainee who becomes effective faster
- a trainee who can be given greater day-to-day responsibility
- a trainee whose morale and self-confidence is high
- a trainee who respects the coach for first-class training.

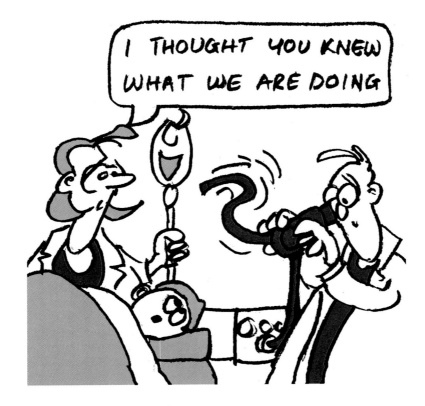

The **responsibilities of the trainee** are:

- a commitment to learning — being motivated
- a willingness to work hard through study and practice
- a responsive attitude to the coach's guidance and advice.

Unless these are evident, the trainee forfeits the right to expect much commitment from the trainer and cannot complain if the coach loses interest. It may not be enough for the trainee to be committed: the trainer has to be shown that this is so — by the trainee taking an active interest in being taught, for example, by going out of his/her way to attend interesting case discussions or ask intelligent questions.

The **rewards for the trainee** are:

- receiving more teaching
- getting better at the job faster
- being trusted by the trainer and so being given more responsibility.

If a trainer is not very interested in training, the trainee may have to take diplomatic action to elicit more or better training — see Section 5, p. 23.

The **partnership between Consultant and Specialist Registrar** is essential to ensure the highest quality training for SHOs. Both play a coaching role, but the allocation of responsibilities should always be as explicit as possible, the roles should be complementary, and the contribution of the Specialist Registrar should remain under the supervision of the Consultant.

The **rewards of such a partnership** are:

- more coherent training of the SHO
- the trainer becomes a more effective coach
- a 'training culture' that fosters learning is created
- the reputation for training leads to better applicants for junior posts.

- **Practise** as much as you can.
  A trainee physician needs constant clinical practice, a coach needs constant coaching practice.

- **Partnership matters**.
  OJT is not something a trainer does to a trainee: it is a joint enterprise in which trainers and trainees cooperate to advance learning. Trainers observe one another coaching and discuss the skills involved. Trainees will give feedback to trainers if invited to do so.

- **Progression** in coaching skills and progression in the knowledge and skills of assessment, diagnosis, and management are both the outcome of practice combined with feedback from partners. In coaching as in medicine, you can't expect to improve without practice and feedback from partners.

4 PROGRESSION IN TRAINING

> Coaching is an integral part of teaching the inexperienced of any age . . . A coaching relationship exists if someone seeks to move someone else along a series of steps, when those steps are not entirely institutionalised and invariant, and when the learner is not entirely clear about their sequence (although the coach is). The coach has to know when to force his man over a hurdle and when to let him sidle up to it . . . The coach may be rejected if he forces too fast a pace, especially at the outset. On the other hand, the pupil . . . may be lost to his mentor if the latter moves too slowly — lost through boredom, shattering of faith or other reasons.
>
> Anselm Strauss, medical sociologist, 1969

THIS SECTION

- **describes the steps of progression in a physician's training**
- **explores how they apply in practice**

Coaching means moving the learner along a series of steps that are clear to the coach but as yet unclear to the trainee. For example, the steps of progression in the acquisition of the competences needed by a physician may be charted in the form of a scheme such as in Diagram 1.

Progression for physicians — a schematic approach

NOVICE →→→→→→→→→→→→→→→→→→→→→→→→→→→→→			EXPERIENCED	
LEVEL ONE	LEVEL TWO	LEVEL THREE	LEVEL FOUR	LEVEL FIVE

←————————— RARE CONDITIONS —————————→

LEVEL THREE	LEVEL FOUR	LEVEL FIVE	beyond
	simple	complex	UNAIDED
simple	complex	WITH HELP	

←————————— UNUSUAL CONDITIONS —————————→

LEVEL TWO	LEVEL THREE	LEVEL FOUR	LEVEL FIVE
	simple	complex	UNAIDED
simple	complex	WITH HELP	

←————————— COMMON CONDITIONS —————————→

LEVEL ONE	LEVEL TWO	LEVEL THREE	LEVEL FOUR
	simple	complex	UNAIDED
simple	complex	WITH HELP	

NOVICE →→→→→→→→→→→→→→→→→→→→→→→→→→→→→			EXPERIENCED	

Conditions (diseases, illnesses) are divided into three categories: common, unusual and rare. They arise in either simple (typical, without complications) or complex (atypical, with complications) form. The trainee can deal with them with or without help. These are then set into a progressive ladder of five levels of increasing competence. Progression means moving in as orderly a way as possible from step to step in a sequence.

At Level 1 the trainee is a novice lacking the ability to assess, diagnose and manage even simple cases of the most common conditions without the help, or under the supervision, of a more senior physician. Many SHOs are in this position on their first day in a specialty. The first and immediate task for such an SHO is to get to Level 2 — being able to deal with simple, common conditions without help, but needing help with more complex cases. At this point the trainee is, under supervision and with help, beginning to deal with simple cases of more unusual conditions. Progression follows this pattern — divided into what is appropriate for a trainee at the various stages of their training. By the point of the Certificate of Completion of Specialist Training (CCST), Specialist Registrars are at Level 4, as are new Consultants. At Level 5 is the highly experienced Consultant who can deal with complex, rare conditions.

The coach aids progression by arranging for learning opportunities that ease the trainee's movement from one step to the next.

The trainee is not at the same level for all aspects. For example, a trainee will be at a higher level with regard to managing a condition than to diagnosing it.

Experienced physicians and trainers have a mental version of a scheme of progression.

> I think the important thing is at that stage, for somebody junior to see how some-body senior appropriately manages a patient. The next stage is to say: 'You go and see this patient, come back and tell me what you would like to do' and then: 'Go and see this patient, I think you should be doing this sort of thing' and then ultimately, 'Go and see this patient, and come and speak to me if there are any particular problems that you are worried about.' So I think gradually taking the individual from being in the swimming pool with them at the shallow end and them being in the deep end on their own swimming free. I think the swimming pool analogy is a very useful one to clinical training.
>
> Trainer

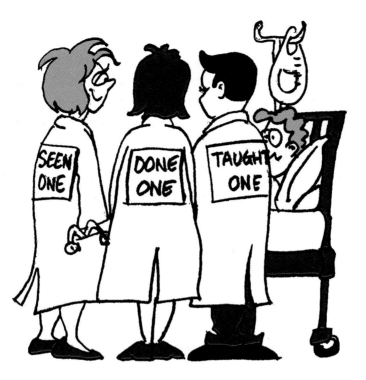

The development of more explicit curricula and the specification of competences, for example, are clarifying what is involved in the staged transition from medical novice to Consultant. (See also Section 13)

New SHOs have, on registration, become competent at a basic level but they are, with regard to the specialist training now to be acquired, once again novices. In the movement from novice to Consultant status, trainees will progress through the levels. Trainees quickly reach higher levels for the simpler tasks, but will be at lower levels for more complex skills.

A trainee is unlikely to pass through the levels at the appropriate rate if the trainer does not actively coach in a systematic way, monitoring carefully the level of the trainee and then judging at what point and in which way the trainee must be moved on. This necessarily includes accurate feedback from coach to trainees (see Section 9), who otherwise may either believe they are not ready to move forward by under-estimating their own competence and achievement, or, by over-estimating their abilities, seek to make progress before they are ready. Monitoring by the coach of trainee over- and under-confidence is a key to ensuring proper progression by trainees.

Specification of the expected competences (knowledge, skills, understanding) to be acquired during each stage of training is probably a precondition of ensuring more efficient and effective progression by trainees — see Section 10 on training plans.

Accurate self-assessment by trainees of their level enhances progression, because it helps to focus trainee learning. The coach takes action either to check whether trainee self-assessment is accurate or to help the trainee develop the skill of accurate self-assessment. The assessments by both partners must be kept aligned.

5 TAKE CONTROL OF YOUR LEARNING

> *By teaching I mean the imparting of knowledge, and for that we are dependent on our teachers; by training I mean the cultivation of aptitude, and for that we are dependent on our opportunities and ourselves.*
>
> Wilfred Trotter, surgeon, 1932
>
> *It is as much the responsibility of the subordinate to manage his [coach] as of the [coach] to manage his subordinate.*
>
> Sir John Harvey-Jones, industrialist, 1994
>
> *Trainees will learn best when they see educational opportunities in every clinical situation.*
>
> The Report of SCOPME, 1994
> (The Standing Committee on Postgraduate Medical Education)

THIS SECTION:

- **explains how, by taking the initiative, you can elicit teaching from your trainer**
- **shows how doing so is a skill you can learn, not a personality characteristic you can't change**
- **illustrates how to take the initiative**

Consultants with trainees, wholly or partly funded by Postgraduate Deans, have an obligation to provide training. Trainees are obliged to be committed to learning and to play an appropriate role as trainee.

In practice, formal obligations and good intentions with regard to training often fall foul of the daily grind. The demands of service on both trainers and trainees frequently distract both parties from the rich possibilities of OJT. Indeed service is always in danger of squeezing out OJT. If trainees view their training passively and assume that the initiative always lies with trainers, then many opportunities for training remain unexploited.

Taking the initiative in your training—what some people call 'being pro-active'—means two things:

- avoiding taking too passive an approach to training
- exploiting fully the potential within service for learning from the cases at hand and the important or subtle differences between them.

23

> At medical school people are spoon-fed a lot of formal teaching but later the onus for training passes onto the trainees to get themselves trained. Although it makes it hard in some sense, it means that some people don't get as much out of the job as they should. Some people are forceful and are more prepared to ask questions or say they don't understand. Other people are shy and retiring, are less assertive and therefore get involved less. It does involve people really using their own initiative to come and get themselves trained.
>
> Trainee

Observation is an important part of learning, but watching an expert may yield only partial understandings. Explanation by the trainer is also necessary to disclose their medical reasoning. Trainers therefore need to explain their clinical decisions and actions. At the same time, trainees need to be prepared to elicit this information from their teachers.

To take control of your learning means:

- taking an active role in shaping training, not passively accepting what is given
- taking the initiative to elicit teaching from trainers, not passively waiting for it
- being ready to ask questions of the trainer, not just answer them
- suggesting possible solutions to problems, not saying 'I don't know what to do'
- keeping your eye open for situations from which you might learn something e.g. an interesting or unusual case
- asking to be present at, and/or participate in, work which is not part of your duty
- bouncing back when taking the initiative has not worked out for you.

Some trainees do these things more naturally or readily than others. One Consultant divided trainees into three kinds:

- those who are diffident and take too little initiative—'the wallflower'
- those who never miss a chance to learn, but do so in a way that does not irritate the coach—the 'fly-trap'
- those who are too pushy and become a nuisance to the trainer—the 'bramble'.

This Section is particularly addressed to trainees who feel that taking the initiative runs against the grain of their personality.

Consider first what trainees themselves say:

'FLY TRAP' TRAINEES WHO TAKE CONTROL

I think the degree [of teaching] you get is dependent on how much enthusiasm you put across. . . At the end of the day, it's like anything. If you're enthusiastic you get taught and you get taught a heck of a lot, but if you're not interested, then people will just wash their hands of you instantly.

Trainees at the diffident end of the spectrum approach training in a very different way:

'WALLFLOWER' TRAINEES

There's a contrast in the department. You can get your way by niggling away at people and that would be one way for me to achieve more training. But that's not the way I see that I should be. Why should I be a nuisance to achieve a goal when my job description is just not being fulfilled?

Some people are more shy, some people are more pushy. The aggressive ones tend to get ahead and the shy ones are left behind. Because they're not coming forward, their shyness is taken as a lack of interest.

I'm quite a diffident person and there were three other juniors with me in the department, so I did tend to miss out on things and I was more or less resorted to as being the suppository putter-inner, whereas what I really wanted was to do the procedure myself with the Consultant watching over my shoulder. I think the other juniors with me were more pushy and they got more out of it than I did.

Such trainees will get more out of their training if they think of taking the initiative not as an unchangeable personality characteristic but as a skill or technique for getting what is rightfully theirs—some solid OJT. Getting the balance right by becoming a 'flytrap' is important for both the wallflowers and the brambles.

'BRAMBLE' TRAINEES

It's pretty irritating, the ones that are constantly questioning everything and are not thinking, but they ask questions for the heck of it. And it's also fairly irritating to have people that are so passive that, you know, you or them are going to fall asleep.

Consultant

Taking the initiative is an aspect of the trainee's partnership with the coach. The professional interaction that takes place between trainees and trainers during ward rounds, or in clinics, provides opportunities for trainees to ask questions, clarifies something the trainee may not yet fully understand or develops deeper knowledge about diseases, treatments, doses or investigations.

Taking control of your learning is not just about getting hands-on experience but shaping the teaching that goes with it.

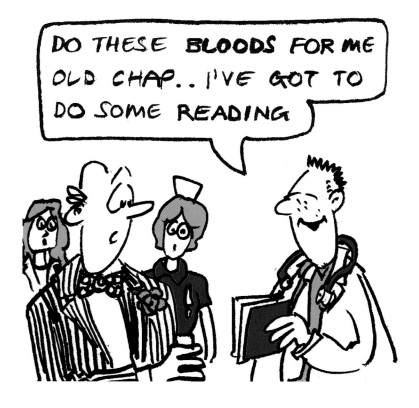

Putting it into action

It does, of course, require a degree of confidence to be pro-active, but it can be done if trainees:

- scan all service for opportunities for training and are ready to seize the initiative
- learn to take the initiative by doing it in small ways where the trainer is almost certain to agree
- take the initiative in matters where they can prove they are ready to be given the responsibility
- choose situations with good chances that a request will be granted, e.g. where there is not too much time pressure on the trainer
- adopt a 'win some, lose some' philosophy and convince themselves they will not feel snubbed or upset if their request is refused.

Trainers help trainees make more of their learning opportunities in OJT when they actively encourage them to take responsibility for their learning and so to be ready to take the initiative in appropriate circumstances. This is a feature of effective coaching. Trainees are better than trainers at spotting training opportunities: it is in their interest to do so, whereas trainers are often deeply engaged in service delivery and so inevitably let some opportunities slip by unnoticed.

Here, we see some of the ways in which a relatively experienced trainee elicits teaching in a pro-active manner:

> In this medical specialty the trainer and the trainee had developed a productive partnership where the trainee had become accustomed to asking questions and giving his medical opinion. Over the file trolley the trainee briefed his trainer but also offered his clinical judgements where he could.
>
> Trainee: *He is more stable than two days ago, but I would certainly want to warfarinise him.*
>
> The trainee shared his ideas and concerns upon which he needed his trainer's views.
>
> Trainee: *Is there something we could have missed? I'm not sure what we might have done differently.*

Whenever the trainer and trainee were walking to another venue or had a few moments to spare, such as when waiting for nursing staff to conclude their care for a patient, the trainee often used this slack time as an opportunity to raise matters he wanted to follow up or check out with his trainer.

Trainee: *I did a literature search on MRSA and the books suggest. . .* [which led to a brief discussion on MRSA].

The most difficult task for the coach is to encourage trainees to take the initiative but without feeling that they are thereby committed to granting all requests. Some requests will and should be refused: it is the style of the refusal, not the refusal itself, that counts. If the refusal is done pleasantly with a clear reason and, wherever possible, an assurance that the request will be granted at a later stage, trainees do not feel dented or diminished and so retreat from taking the initiative in future.

ACTION POINTS ON BEING PRO-ACTIVE

TRAINEES

- be active in shaping your training and eliciting teaching from your coach(es)
- aim to be a 'fly-trap'. Avoid the extremes of being too diffident ('wallflower') and too pushy ('bramble')
- scan all service for opportunities for teaching and learning
- ask to do things, but make sure you're ready for the responsibility
- don't worry if some of your requests are refused
- suggest to your coach solutions to your problems—you learn more than simply asking for advice about what to do.

TRAINERS

- encourage trainees, especially those who seem diffident, to take the initiative in promoting teaching and learning
- create the conditions under which trainees accept responsibility for taking control of their training
- ensure that taking the initiative pays off for the trainee
- tell trainees in what matters or on what occasions taking the initiative is not welcome
- avoid snubbing behaviour where a request is inappropriate in content or timing
- refuse trainee requests sometimes, but never humiliate
- accept that a good trainee will be impatient to progress and so will be eager for more responsibility or experience.

6   HOW TO ASK QUESTIONS (1)

> *Question asking is the royal road to knowledge and learning.*
> Seymour Sarason, psychologist, 1993
>
> *The seeker for knowledge will profit from guide-ropes and tug-ropes.*
> William Evans, physician, 1968

THIS SECTION

- **shows why questioning is a key skill in coaching**
- **explains the forms and functions of questions**
- **focuses on questions that stimulate thinking and reasoning**
- **suggests how to develop your questioning skills**

Questioning is under-used as a technique in medical OJT, and it is a more subtle skill than many coaches realise. Training is better if there is more questioning and it is done more skilfully.

FOR TRAINEES

This Section is largely designed for coaches, and shows how to question you in a way that helps you to learn effectively. You should look through this Section to understand fully when some kinds of questioning can sometimes be challenging, even painful, if you are to be stretched to the full.

What is a question? What's the point of asking questions? How and why do they contribute to learning?

Questions take different **forms** and serve different **functions** and have variable **value** for training. Consider how these three ideas work in practice.

There are two basic forms of question—open and closed.

Closed questions have a known and fixed answer which is clearly either right or wrong.

e.g. What does DVT stand for?

Open questions have several possible or plausible answers or, sometimes, no obvious or uncontentious answer at all.

e.g. *What prophylactic measures can be used to prevent DVT?*

Other questions can be answered simply by a 'yes' or 'no' and so are neither obviously open nor closed. If a yes or no is sufficient as a competent answer requiring no further justification or elaboration, then the question is half-closed.

Question: *Can subcutaneous heparin be used to prevent DVT?*

Answer: *Yes.*

If the response of yes or no is not an adequate answer and the questioner can reasonably expect some elaboration, then the question is **half-open**.

Question: *Is subcutaneous heparin the best prophylaxis against DVT?*

Answer: *Yes, because . . .*

Here are some examples of questions asked of trainees by trainers. Can you say which are open, closed, half-open and half-closed? Which have the greatest value for helping the trainee to learn?

- *what do we call this type of infection?*
- *which cranial nerve does this?*
- *do you know how to classify leukaemias?*
- *does this barium enema show a stenosis?*
- *would you inject this joint?*
- *how does this chest X-ray help you?*
- *why do you think this ulcer will not heal?*
- *how could you tell if there is an underlying tumour?*
- *what options are there for management?*
- *under what circumstances would you do a lumbar puncture?*
- *how do you decide whether to give thyroxine or not?*

Closed questions require relatively lower order cognitive functioning, often simple recall. They are appropriate to aspects of medical training, as when the trainer checks that trainees know the relevant physiology. Trainees may be reluctant to answer a closed question unless they are absolutely sure they know the right answer, for to give the wrong answer potentially invites ridicule or censure or even the dreaded public humiliation. Admitting one does not know reveals one's ignorance. The best bet, especially when the question is being asked in a group of trainees, is to say nothing and hope somebody else takes the risk—and so teaching and learning are hindered.

Most closed questions asked by trainers are **test questions**, the function of which is to uncover whether trainees have the relevant knowledge and can give a clear answer—'I know and I want to know if you know'. The limitation of closed questions is that if a trainee provides the right answer, this informs the coach, which can be useful, but it does relatively little for the trainee. It may make the trainee feel good to be able to supply the answer, but no additional learning is taking place. If the answer is wrong, then many trainers respond by providing the right answer. This may help the trainee, but it may not change the faulty reasoning or knowledge that lies behind the wrong answer. Genuine learning means changing the underlying reasoning not just parroting an isolated right answer.

Open questions are usually of a different order, for they demand higher cognitive functions—processes of reasoning, judgement and decision making—and so contribute more to professional learning. Open questions are good in helping trainees develop problem-solving skills.

In a series of closed questions, the trainer is doing most of the asking and telling and the trainee is (the trainer hopes) learning by listening. In a series of open questions, it is the trainee who does most of the talking in having to give a thought-through response to the questions. The coach, by asking good questions, forces the trainee to think. The coach then monitors each response with a view to asking further questions or making supportive comments that will help the trainee arrive at a sound solution or conclusion. Trainees may groan at open questions because of the work that has to be done to sort out an answer, but to the coach the groan is the sign that learning is probably taking place.

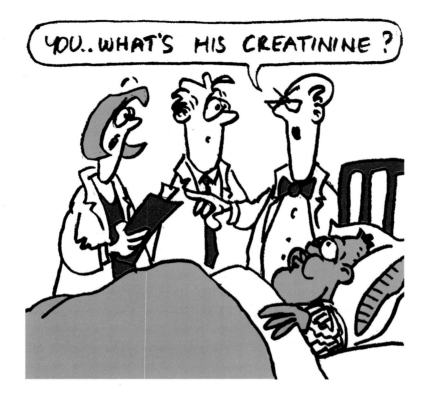

Questioning style

The style of the question can also be very influential. For example, if the trainer poses the question in an aggressive manner, trainees may be so nervous about failing to get the right answer (to a closed question) or about exploring possibilities (to an open question) that no answer is attempted at all. Of course there are times when a question should be challenging, and trainees are more likely to respond if the question is put gently with an explicit statement that the question is a tough one. Coaches push a trainee hard through questions, but the manner adopted is carefully fitted to the character of the trainee and the nature of the occasion.

Being challenging does not require the coach to be aggressive or oppressive.

> There is nothing worse than being cut down in public in front of your House Officer and patients: . . . that is deeply demoralising and then there is no point in being pro-active.
>
> Trainee
>
> [I know] only too well one has to be very careful not to humiliate or insult the trainee in front of other colleagues and patients because it destroys everyone's relationship with each other.
>
> Trainer

Coaches always remember that trainees are far more conscious than the coach of the nature of the audience who are witnessing any response from trainees: no trainee likes to be made to look foolish or inappropriately ignorant before peers, nurses or patients. Public humiliation is not a sound teaching technique.

> There are ways of answering questions, even if they are 'stupid'. You can emphasise its stupidity to everyone around or simply answer the question but make it apparent to the individual that really the answer was obvious.
>
> Trainer

Questioning to evoke higher order thinking and reasoning

In asking questions, the coach can have very different functions in mind—to get the trainee to hypothesise about possible causes; to speculate about effects; to reach a decision; to solve a problem. Asking open rather than closed questions can be more effective in getting the trainee to engage in the necessary, and sometimes painful, higher order thinking.

Examine the examples overleaf. Do the open questions stimulate higher order thinking more effectively?

A closed question is often answered quickly, since trainees either know or they don't. Silence usually means that nobody knows the answer. Open questions, because they demand much more thought, are often not answered quickly and silence often means simply that trainees are thinking. A glance at trainees' faces will usually indicate to the coach whether silence reflects thinking or bewilderment.

HIGHER ORDER QUESTIONS

1. To get the trainee to identify and hypothesise about the character and causes of a condition
   - What's wrong with this patient? [Closed]
   - How has this condition come about in this patient? [Open]

2. To get the trainee to identify and hypothesise about the effects and consequences of treatment
   - What does the book say the effects of this drug are? [Closed]
   - D'you realise what will happen if you do that? [Half-closed]
   - What would happen to the patient if you . . .? [Open]

3. To encourage trainee decision making
   - What's the right way to treat this? [Closed]
   - What are the options for managing this condition? [Open]

4. To help the trainee with problem solving
   - Do you know how to solve this? [Half-closed]
   - Can you think of ways of solving this? [Half-open]
   - How might you get round that difficulty? [Open]

5. To help the trainee to evaluate a decision or conclusion
   - Did you make the right decision? [Half-closed]
   - How will you know if that was a good decision? [Open]

Trainers need to learn to leave a decent pause for this **thinking time**—at least 5 seconds. If the coach steps in too quickly—and most trainers do—thinking is interrupted and discouraged. It takes an effort for the coach to remain silent during this critical thinking time. Remember: the better the question, the longer the thinking time you allow. The silence that follows a good question is hard for the trainer to tolerate, but not for the trainees.

Even so, a trainee will sometimes come up with a poor answer. The temptation for the coach may then be to step in with a correctional statement which provides a better answer. A more effective way of helping the trainee to learn is to ask another open question. This either helps the trainee towards a better answer or exposes the reasoning behind the poor answer. To correct the reasoning behind a faulty answer is better teaching than to correct the faulty answer itself.

Compare the following two exchanges between trainee and trainer. The first is short and snappy: the second takes much longer. Both cover the same topic. Is one a better piece of teaching than the other? What reasons can you suggest to defend your answer? Can another point of view be defended?

Exchange 1

Trainer   *Why do we take blood cultures in a patient with septicaemia?*

Trainee   *To know which antibiotics to prescribe.*

Trainer   *No, the results take 48 hours. It is to make sure that the organisms are sensitive to the antibiotics prescribed.*

Now consider this longer exchange.

Exchange 2

Trainer   *Why do we take blood cultures in a patient with septicaemia?*

Trainee   *To know which antibiotics to prescribe.*

Trainer   *How long do the results usually take to come back?*

Trainee   *You sometimes get a preliminary report after 24 hours and a full report after 48 hours.*

Trainer   *So how do you choose which antibiotics to give when you first see the patient?*

Trainee   *You decide on the most likely organisms present according to the presumed source of the infection.*

Trainer   *And then?*

Trainee   *And you then choose the most appropriate antibiotics to which the organisms are most likely to be sensitive. A best-guess therapy.*

Trainer   *So what do you ask the microbiologist when she phones the following day?*

Trainee   *What organisms are growing in the blood cultures that I took?*

Trainer   *And?*

Trainee   *And if they are sensitive to the antibiotics that I have prescribed?*

Trainer   *So why do we take the blood cultures?*

Trainee   *It is to check that the organisms are sensitive to the antibiotics prescribed.*

Trainer   *Well done!*

So to develop your questioning skills, follow these four rules of thumb.

FOUR RULES OF THUMB FOR QUESTIONING

- **Restrict closed questions to test questions.** They are appropriate when you want to know whether the trainee knows something factual.

- **Ask open questions in all other circumstances.** They are more likely to stimulate the higher order cognitive processes essential to learning beyond merely committing to memory.

- **Allow adequate thinking time** after an open question—at least 5 seconds.

- **Follow a poor answer with an open question.** It will lead to the trainee changing direction, or expose the faulty reasoning behind the wrong answer.

In everyday situations we do not think about the question we want to ask, then take time to decide what its best form and function might be, and finally actually ask it. Rather, we formulate the question in a particular way whilst we are thinking it out—the formulation and the asking often occur simultaneously in a kind of 'thinking out loud'.

Questions in semi-formal sessions

Learning how to question takes time. Fortunately there are plenty of opportunities for practising the art. Many medical departments have some form of regular meeting at which team members brief each other about their patients and/or recent admissions and decisions on management. These are essentially business meetings, but are often and quite naturally transformed into occasions for semi-formal teaching. In other words, for service reasons the trainer asks test questions to check trainee knowledge and then diverges from the real cases at hand to discuss wider issues arising from the case. Sometimes this is done in response to a question from the trainee. Questions, then, are a natural part of semi-formal sessions.

Can the number of questions asked, either by coaches or trainees, be increased to enhance OJT in these sessions?

In a typical, daily meeting of this kind, lasting for 30 minutes or so, the trainer will, with no special or self-conscious intention, ask half a dozen questions which serve a teaching function. This adds up to 30 questions a week or 1,500 a year. Such a bank of questions is evidently a powerful teaching device. The questioning rate is around one question for every 5 minutes. If this rate can be doubled from 6 to 12—an easy target to achieve if you try it for yourself—it means, of course, another 1,500 questions a year. With a relatively small effort, the OJT element in a naturally occurring semi-formal occasion can be dramatically strengthened.

Of course the quality of the question is important too. Here are some guides to aid your practice. Do not try to use all four on any one occasion. Try one at a time. Once you feel comfortable with each, you will find yourself able to use more than one in a single OJT session.

Ask one good question every time

One question that really tells is more effective than a lot of poor ones—and saves time too. So if you know you're going to question trainees about a topic, ahead of time think up one really good question that will set them thinking, and make sure you put it. With practice, you'll find it easier to think up good questions on the spot.

Practise one type of higher order question

It's not easy to learn to ask, on a consistent basis, the open, higher order questions described above. So practise them one at a time. In one session, decide to focus on one type—questions about causes, or questions about effects and consequences, or questions about decisions, and so on.

Use the counter-question

In other words, respond to a question with a further question. *How shall I manage this patient?* asks the trainee. *What do you see as the options?* counters the coach. This makes the trainee think and informs the coach about the level and quality of the trainee's knowledge and thinking on the topic. It also gives the coach space to think about possible answers too.

Nominate the trainee to answer

If you rely on volunteers to answer, some trainees will volunteer much more frequently than others. By sometimes nominating the person to answer you make sure those who are shy still get a fair share of the questions and an opportunity to participate. You also keep everyone on their toes. People tend to pay more attention if they think there is a chance that they will be called on to answer.

Role reversals—getting trainees to ask questions

Most question-and-answer sessions are trainer-led—the trainer asks the questions and the trainees provide (some of) the answers. As we have seen, there is a danger that the coach ends up asking mostly test questions, which do little to promote learning. It is the trainees who are sometimes best placed to know what they do not know or understand, so learning can be increased if roles can be reversed—trainees ask the questions and the coach answers.

Trainers often say they would like this to happen, but trainees don't seem keen to ask questions. Almost always this is because the coach has not used the best method for making trainees feel comfortable about asking questions. This approach will discourage trainees from asking questions.

> *OK. Any questions?* (One second pause). *Jolly good. Back to work!*

And so will these responses if you do get a question.

> *If you'd been listening to what I've been saying, you'd know the answer to that.*

or

> *Don't they teach anything at all in medical schools these days?*

Getting trainees to ask questions for their own sake is pointless. However trainees often do have questions but are nervous about asking them in case they end up looking stupid or inattentive or even ingratiating. So most trainees' questions remain unanswered because they never get asked.

A good coach makes room for questions and invites trainees to fill the space provided. To encourage trainees to feel free to ask questions, try these alternative approaches.

> *OK. That was quite a difficult topic and I expect some of you have questions. Who'd like to ask the first one?* Count 5 seconds—only you will feel at all uncomfortable in the short silence—and if there's still no question, say: *Are there parts of what I said that seem at all unclear or difficult to follow that we might usefully go through?*

Trainees often take up such secondary invitations, because they have had sufficient space to think it out. If a question is asked, support the asking:

> *Mm. That's a good question. Now . . .*

or

> *I was hoping someone would raise that because . . .*

Sometimes a trainee will put a question in a very short and tentative form. By smart use of a counter-question, the coach gets the trainee to develop the question or move to an answer, thus making the trainee do more of the learning work. For example, try:

- **the counter-question for clarification**—*Good question. Do you mean. . .?* where the trainee did not mean that, and so talks further to clarify what was intended—which informs the coach about trainee thinking.
- **the counter-question for elaboration** —*That's interesting, but aren't you raising the issue of. . .?* which encourages the trainee to set the question in a wider context and make new connections.
- **the counter-question for role reversal**—*Good question: do you want to make a stab at what an answer might be?*—trainees often know more than they think they know.

> The clever thing about my trainer's approach to training me is that he answers questions by asking me questions. Instead of giving me a simple answer, he talks me through it. It's more active learning for me.
>
> Trainee

ACTION POINTS ON QUESTIONING

TRAINERS
- ask open questions whenever you can
- ask higher order questions whenever you can:
  - — to hypothesise about the sources/causes of a condition
  - — to hypothesise about the effects/consequences of a condition
  - — to engage in problem-solving
  - — to encourage decision making
  - — to evaluate a conclusion or decision
- allow thinking time for open questions—5 seconds—the better the question, the longer the thinking time needed
- ask challenging questions gently and slowly
- don't 'put down' a trainee who asks a question that seems stupid
- ask closed questions only to test trainee knowledge
- follow a poor answer with another question
- use questions to reveal and develop trainee reasoning
- get trainees to ask more of their own questions:
  - —by allowing time for trainees to think out their questions
  - —by making them feel comfortable about asking questions
  - —by approving good questions
  - —by asking counter-questions as your answer
- ask more questions in the semi-formal meetings you hold.

7 HOW TO ASK QUESTIONS (II)

> Questioning is a far more difficult form of pedagogy for teachers than telling, because it is the least predictable.
>
> Theodore Sizer, educationist, 1984

THIS SECTION:
- **explains how to ask double questions**
- **explains how to turn closed into open sequences**
- **explains how to engage in holistic questioning**
- **explains how to reformulate *why?* questions.**

These four skills are easy to explain but harder to put into practice.

Asking double questions

When questioning, you may find it helps to do a little double questioning. One common problem is realising that, after you have asked a question, its form is less than ideal. A way round this is to follow on with a second question which reformulates the first, thus making a double question.

You can double question in other circumstances too. For instance, when you get no reply from the trainee to your first question, reformulate it into a version more likely to elicit a response.

The are four common types of double question.

1. REFORMULATE CLOSED TO OPEN

Here the coach asks a double question to get round the problem of having asked an initial closed question. Recognising this, the coach immediately reformulates it in a open form.

- *What is the way to treat a pneumothorax? What options are there?*

Trainees tend to respond to the last version of a question, and in this case the reformulated open version is educationally preferable.

43

2. REFORMULATE OPEN TO CLOSED

This is useful when there is no response to the original open question and, for reasons of time pressure or the difficulty of the question, the coach wants a quick response.

- *Where do you think the block is in this patient's coronary arteries?* [Silence] *Is it in the right or the left?*

- *What can you say about this patient's swollen legs?* [Silence] *Is there cellulitis or thrombosis?*

3. REFORMULATE FOR CLARIFICATION

The first question may be reformulated in a simpler or clearer form to help the trainees, who generally are unwilling to say they don't fully understand the question or see the point of it.

- *Do you think the drain is in position? Is the water level in the drain swinging with breathing?*

4. A NUDGING DOUBLE QUESTION

Another use of double questioning to support learning is to use the second question as a means of gently nudging trainees into a response. The second question may contain a clue or hint, which serves as 'scaffolding' to push trainee thinking and reasoning forward beyond what they think they know.

- *Is this going to work? Do you think this diuretic will be strong enough?*

- *What is the management of this patient? Have you any of the latest ideas?*

- *What does this patient need for therapy? What types of thrombolysis do you know?*

- *What does this ECG show? Are there any ST segment changes?*

Questions in sequence

The way we think about questions most of the time is that they occur naturally as one of a pair, that is, a question is linked to, and usually followed by, an answer.

In a teaching context, questions have a more complicated structure and usually occur as the first element in a triplet, not a pair. This is because the trainer asks the question; the trainee answers; and then the trainer has an extra turn in evaluating the answer. Consider the following exchanges.

Exchange 1

First speaker: *What time is it?*

Second speaker: *One o'clock.*

First speaker: *Yes, that's right. Well done!*

Exchange 2

First speaker: *What time is it?*

Second speaker: *Two o'clock.*

First speaker: *No, it's one o'clock.*

If in everyday circumstances we asked somebody for the time, we would be astounded to be congratulated on our answer or have it corrected or be told it despite our ignorance [Exchange 1]. This is because we assume the questioner is making an enquiry to which he or she does not already know the answer [Exchange 2].

The first triplet makes sense only if the first speaker is teaching the second speaker how to tell the time. This is evident from the first speaker's second turn, which is either an acceptance through praise or a correction of an error. In a teaching situation the participants assume that the teacher does know the answer to the question and is asking not to obtain information but to test whether the trainee knows as well.

Closed sequences

Questions with a clear, factual answer are usually closed questions, which often appear as the opening move in a triplet. At the end of the triplet, the trainer moves naturally to asking another closed question, so that the teaching takes the form of **closed triplets in a sequence.**

45

Trainer:	*Closed question 1*
Trainee:	*Answer or statement of ignorance*
Trainer:	*Acceptance/correction/answer supplied*
Trainer:	*Closed question 2*
Trainee:	*Answer or statement of ignorance*
Trainer:	*Acceptance/correction/answer supplied*

and so on.

There is nothing wrong with asking closed questions, but it is evident that the trainee is not doing much learning here but merely rehearsing existing knowledge for the benefit of the trainer. If the trainee gets most of the answers right, it is the trainer who does most of the learning—learning that the trainee is not very ignorant!

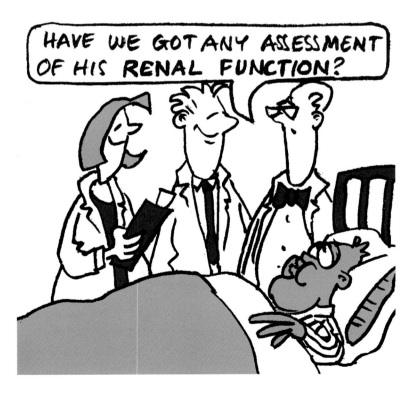

Open sequences

More active trainee learning occurs when the coach turns a sequence into an open one. This is done by asking an open question, so that we get an open triplet of the following form.

Coach: *Question—open or closed*

Trainee: *Answer*

Coach: *Open question*

Consider the following examples.

Open triplet example 1

Coach: *How should we manage this patient?*

Trainee: *I don't know*

Coach: *What options do you think there are?*

The coach does not supply the missing answer, but by using the open counter-question forces the trainee to think, which may well reveal that the trainee has some inkling of what good management might be.

Open triplet example 2

Coach: *How should we manage this patient?*

Trainee: *With chemotherapy.*

Coach: *Are there circumstances when palliative treatment is indicated?*

Here the coach avoids the premature 'closure' that is created by accepting or correcting the answer. Through another open question, the trainee is pressed to think out exceptions which will reveal the true extent of understanding. The trainee may finally be told that the first answer was 'right', but their learning has been extended.

Turning closed triplets into open triplets is a relatively easy way of making the trainee learn in a deep rather than a superficial way.

Open triplet example 3

Coach: *How should we manage this patient?*

Trainee: *Using drug therapy*

Coach: *Do you think that is better than physiotherapy?*

The coach declines the expected last turn of a closed triplet and neither accepts nor corrects the trainee's answer. The trainee is distracted from looking for a 'right or wrong' response and is pushed by the extra open question into setting the answer within the framework of a larger question. The trainer has initiated some holistic questioning (each answer being logically related to other answers which, taken as a whole, form a reasoned argument) in place of atomistic questioning, or questions and answers only loosely related to one another with no coherent overall argument.

Holistic *versus* atomistic questioning

Let us consider a real case. A trainee briefs her trainer about a new admission.

This is a 51 year old woman who is a known schizophrenic, who, this morning at the railway station, had a fit, a generalised seizure lasting 5 minutes, which was preceded by an episode of panic, although this wasn't associated with any physical symptoms. During the seizure, she was incontinent of urine and bit her tongue. This was witnessed by her partner. On arriving in A&E, she was slightly drowsy, GCS [Glasgow Coma Scale] 15 and on examination there was nothing remarkable to find except that her O_2 saturation was 90% on air. The gases suggested that she was slightly hypoxic, ECG was normal, chest X-ray looks normal. Why did she have a fit and what do I do with her?

The following discussion between the trainer and trainee then took place.

> Trainer: So what do you think's going on with this woman?
> Trainee: I think she's obviously had a seizure for some reason, which I think is probably related to the hypoxia, that's the only thing that's abnormal that I can find.
> Trainer: So what do her gases show?
> Trainee: Her gases show that she's slightly acidotic, slightly hypoxic and that her carbon dioxide's slightly raised but not significantly.
> Trainer: So she's got—?
> Trainee: She's got a respiratory acidosis.

Trainer:	Yes. With—?
Trainee:	Mild with compensation.
Trainer:	Yes. OK. And her pH is normal, so she's almost normal, so she's compensating. What's her oxygen?
Trainee:	Her oxygen is 9.18. That's low.
Trainer:	So she's—?
Trainee:	Hypoxic.
Trainer:	OK. And is that on air?
Trainee:	Yes.
Trainer:	So that's abnormal?
Trainee:	Yes.
Trainer:	Excellent. So are there any other signs or symptoms to find on examination?
Trainee:	On listening to the chest, she has slightly decreased air entry at the right base and looking at that, I'm slightly, I don't know — she isn't taking very big breaths inwards; it might be a slightly raised right hemi-diaphragm.
Trainer:	And on the chest X-ray?
Trainee:	The shadowing might be a little bit abnormal as well. Could be some consolidation or fluid on that side of the chest.
Trainer:	Any other investigations that you've done?
Trainee:	Yes, an ECG which was normal. And I've done blood tests, U's and E's, full blood count, glucose.
Trainer:	Good.
Trainee:	And that's it.
Trainer:	Are there any other findings on the chest X-ray that you think are abnormal that you haven't mentioned already?
Trainee:	A slightly deviated trachea, I thought, just now. [She points at something else on the X-ray at this point]
Trainer:	OK; what's that mark there?
Trainee:	I'm not sure. I don't know what that is.
Trainer:	Do you think it's normal or abnormal?
Trainee:	Abnormal.
Trainer:	OK. So how do you think that mark fits in with what you've said so far? In a patient who's hypoxic, who's got . . .?
Trainee:	Unless that's an area of infarct?
Trainer:	Well it could be, couldn't it? Or there's another thing called linear atelectasis, which is linear collapse, but that mark there certainly could be an infarct, secondary to—?
Trainee:	A pulmonary embolus.
Trainer:	OK. And the pulmonary embolus would explain—?
Trainee:	The gases.
Trainer:	The gases. OK. And if she's had a PE that would explain—?
Trainee:	Her fit.

> Trainer: *Her fit. OK? So the idea is here that maybe her fit was secondary to the pulmonary embolus, rather than the fit being the primary event and the gases being secondary to the fit, in that she had probably had a PE first and then had a fit secondary to the hypoxia. Does that seem right?*
> Trainee: *Yes.*
> Trainer: *So I think what we should do now is—?*
> Trainee: *Refer her to the medics.*
> Trainer: *Refer her to the medics. Excellent!*

After the trainee's opening question, the trainer could easily have said, quite simply, 'No, she's had a secondary fit to some other cause' and continued the conversation with appropriate further investigations and management. Instead, he decides to make this a piece of teaching in which from the very beginning he sets himself the dual task of:

- uncovering the faulty reasoning behind the trainee's belief that the patient has had a simple, primary, epileptic fit

- getting into place the correct reasoning by which the trainee would understand why the fit is secondary to some other cause.

His first step, therefore, is to avoid giving a quick-fix answer to the question and so instead he offers a counter-question to elicit from the trainee the diagnostic reasoning. He then proceeds to take the trainee through the investigations and findings, getting her to point out the abnormalities so that she sees the flaw in her initial assessment and comes to a full and correct diagnosis and management plan.

The time taken for this exchange is 3 minutes. The trainee has, however, probably learned a great deal since, through questioning, the faulty reasoning has been elicited, then subverted, and finally replaced by correct reasoning. The coach asks many questions, but they are not isolated but simply follow one after the other; they are held together in a holistic way by the overall intention to elicit and correct the trainee's reasoning.

Holistic questioning is rare; it is a difficult skill to master, since there has to be self-control by the coach to avoid sliding into a simple telling of the correct answer;

practice is essential to keep an overall intention of eliciting faulty reasoning; getting the trainee to recognise why it is faulty, before working together to replace it—one hopes permanently—with the right reasoning.

Transforming *why?* questions from trainees

Eliciting the reasoning behind trainee thinking or action is often achieved by a coach through a *why?* question. Indeed, this is the most common way in which trainers demand explanations from trainees.

> *Why did you . . . ?*
> *Why would you . . . ?*
> *Why do you think . . . ?*
> *Why did that happen . . . ?*
> *Why is the patient . . . ?*
> *Why are you managing the patient like that?*

Why? questions are easy to ask: whenever one does not understand, the obvious step is to ask *why?* But *why?* questions have two serious weaknesses:

- they can be very threatening to trainees, putting them immediately on the defensive, which inhibits deep thinking
- they are highly ambiguous.

And the ambiguity increases the sense of threat.

Why? can mean . . .

- what is your intention when you . . . ?
- what is your goal when you . . . ?
- what motivated you when you . . . ?
- what reason do have for doing . . . ?
- what is the logical status of your thinking?
- what is the causal chain involved here?
- what processes are at work here?

- what effects do you hope to achieve?
- what consequences will follow?

Whilst the coach usually has a specific version of the *why?* question in mind, this is buried inside the generality of the *why?*, so the trainee has the double problem of trying to work out what the *why?* really means and the answer to it.

The solution is eminently simple: avoid *why?* questions and be more specific about what you mean. However, it's not easy to get out of the habit of asking sloppy *why?* questions. When you find yourself slipping into one, try the expedient of the **double question**. You hear yourself ask a *why?* question, so immediately reformulate it into a more specific version.

REFORMULATED *WHY?* QUESTIONS

Why are you putting an intravenous line in? What will you gain by using the intravenous route?

Why are you using that new drug? What are the benefits from the new drug as compared to the old one?

Why are you requesting another chest X-ray? What are you hoping to find on a further chest film?

Why are you repeating the blood tests? What further information will you get from repeat blood tests?

Another way in which the coach can learn to reformulate *why?* questions is to ask trainees to clarify any *why?* question they ask—which also has the advantage of making it more likely that any answer the coach gives will meet the trainee's intention in asking the question in the first place.

FURTHER ACTION POINTS ON QUESTIONING

TRAINERS

- use double questions to help trainees answer your questions
  - — reformulate unintended closed questions as open ones
  - — reformulate difficult open questions as closed ones
  - — reformulate to clarify a question
  - — reformulate by hint or clue to 'scaffold' trainee learning
- avoid sequences of closed questions—break them by open questions
- practise the art of holistic questioning, but make sure that trainees see the point of a long sequence of questions and don't lose the thread
- take care with *why?* questions—reformulate to make the purpose behind your question as specific as you can.

8 HOW TO TELL AND EXPLAIN

> *The professional may find it difficult to admit that, although he knows he is successful, he does not know how to tell others how to behave equally effectively.*
>
> Chris Argyris & Donald Schön, educationists, 1974

> *It is invaluable for young trainees to see…into the mental processes of an experienced clinician.*
>
> Lord Walton, former President, Royal Society of Medicine, 1993

> *Oral narrative is a neglected medium for the transmission of medical knowledge. Anecdotes are an informal extension of the case presentations, intended to improve clinical judgement.*
>
> Kathryn M Hunter, medical educator, 1991

THIS SECTION:

- **describes different kinds of telling**
- **shows how telling can be linked with questioning**
- **explains how to use questions to get feedback on telling**

The common form of teaching is telling or explaining—what is often loosely called didactic teaching. A lecture is simply a formal and extended version of this method. Mini-versions of the lecture, **the lecturette,** are used by trainers on ward rounds and in clinics, but they rarely last for more than a few minutes.

More common is the making of **occasional comments** which

- describe what the trainer is thinking or doing
- explain why the trainer is thinking or doing it
- give background information to the description or explanation
- are relevant anecdotes, cautionary tales, jokes and funny stories.

Quite often these are somewhat random and have no very obvious rationale. Effective trainers match the content and style of their comments quite closely to the needs and experience of the trainee. This is much harder to do than it sounds.

55

A very inexperienced trainee will benefit if the coach gives an overall view of the condition and then gives a mixture of description and explanation from time to time to maintain the interest and attention of the trainee, who will otherwise soon become bored or continue to observe but without significant learning. A brief overview of what has been achieved can also be helpful.

Experienced trainees may need little in the way of description and explanation, but will have their needs met if the coach invites them to ask questions whenever they want to. Asking the inexperienced to ask questions whenever they wish is poor strategy, for they either don't know what questions to ask and so keep silent and learn little, or they ask questions all the time, which is irritating and distracting.

Both trainers and trainees give explanations. Trainers usually offer explanations, either on their own initiative or in response to questions from trainees, but trainees usually only respond with explanations because the coach has asked for one.

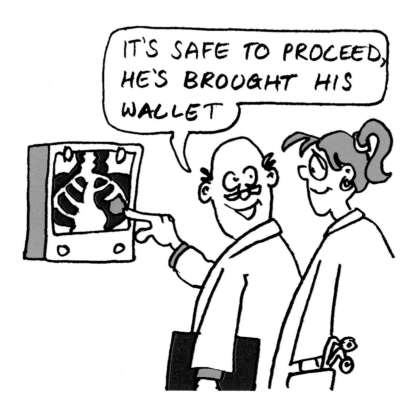

A related but rarely used method is the **running commentary**, when the coach offers a continuous flow of description and explanation. For the physician the running commentary is particularly appropriate for use with teaching procedural skills.

> [It is] particularly useful because the alternatives are either a lecture-based, didactic explanation of how to do a procedure, or just getting on with it. The logical middle step is to be shown one, talked through it and then to actually do one whilst being supervised. That certainly gets rid of a lot of anxiety when you come to do the first one by yourself. I can't see how else you can necessarily teach somebody safely and so that they have a degree of confidence without doing it in that manner. Mannequins are one thing, but doing it on real patients whilst being supervised is so much better.
>
> Trainee
>
> There's only so much that any individual trainee can take in from a certain procedure at any one time and to observe and have some running commentary is good; then there should be a chance to talk through it.
>
> Trainer

A few trainers who are highly experienced can do this, but most can sustain the commentary only for relatively short periods of time. In the more difficult cases, when the physician has to concentrate, a lapse into silence is natural—but for the experienced novice this is the very moment when a commentary from the coach is particularly valuable.

> There should be a chance for the person who undertook the procedure to tell you all those things that he or she did automatically.
>
> Trainer
>
> The complications of a simple procedure aren't always given a running commentary, nor are they given completely.
>
> Trainer

Even more rare is the **thinking out loud** approach, where the coach makes no attempt to judge what the trainee needs by way of description or explanation but simply tries to put into words the mind's content in a stream-of-consciousness style. This again is difficult to do in a sustained way for two main reasons: one's

57

hands can do things more quickly than any verbal account of the action; and many of the things one does are so automatic that the knowledge of how to do it has become 'tacit' or below the level of ordinary consciousness. Despite these difficulties, 'thinking out loud' can be very helpful to trainees in giving insight into the way experienced physicians approach their work. In particular it can give insights into the process of decision making and the factors that influence the making of decisions—something that is often obscured from the trainee relying exclusively on observation of the physician at work.

Specialist Registrars and newly appointed Consultants sometimes find it easier to think out loud because they have acquired the skill more recently and the knowledge has not yet become entirely tacit. If you find that you are good at giving the running commentary or thinking-out-loud—some people are, some are not—then you might try to encourage your trainees to do it too. It may help them to think about what they are doing and it may give you some insight into what and how they are thinking. But don't try to force trainees to do this if they are uncomfortable with it. And remember that many people find thinking-out-loud and the running commentary particularly onerous and distracting when they are concentrating very hard on something they find difficult to do.

Telling with questioning—the didactic *versus* the socratic

Telling, especially describing and explaining, sometimes called the 'didactic' method, is often frowned upon as a teaching method, on the assumption that the so-called 'socratic' methods of teaching-by-questioning is inherently superior. Yet the various forms of telling play a vital role in training, even though, unlike questioning, they do not always exert much pressure on the trainee to engage in active thinking. The best training talk is a careful blend of telling and questioning according to the circumstances.

Uninterrupted telling always risks a lapse of attention in the listening trainees— some of whom are skilled in the art of looking as if they are listening when they are not. Telling is easily 'chunked' or segmented by the insertion of questions at regular intervals. There are two types of question that are helpful here.

The first is the **test question**, discussed in Section 7, which is often a closed question serving to uncover or check the trainee's existing knowledge.

Do you know about. . .?

Are you familiar with. . .?

Have I ever explained about. . .?

What is. . .?

If you don't bother to ask, most trainees are reluctant to tell you that they do know or that you have already told them and so will politely listen to your redundant telling and explaining. At the same time a silence in response to *Do you know...?* and *Are you familiar with...?* types of question often masks a negative—the trainees don't like to acknowledge their ignorance. So a silent response may usefully be followed with a further test question along the lines of *Good, then you'll be able to tell me...* Often trainees then find themselves quite unable to tell the trainer about what they claimed they knew, so there is an opportunity for the trainer pleasantly to remind the trainees that ignorance is no crime and that they should not be embarrassed about revealing it.

The second is the **check out question,** which checks out whether the trainee is understanding or following what you are telling.

Is that clear?

Do you see that?

Are you following me?

OK?

Such questions also have the useful effect of maintaining the listeners' attention to your talk.

A particularly effective sequence is the **explaining triad** which is a sequence of three moves as follows:

- test questions $\longrightarrow$
- explanation, interspersed with check out questions $\longrightarrow$
- more questions to test or to further trainee understanding.

In other words, the coach, instead of proceeding with a long piece of telling:

- first asks one or more **test questions** to ascertain the state of the trainee's knowledge or understanding, thus avoiding the danger of redundant telling
- in the light of the gaps revealed, provides an explanation
- uses regular **check out questions** designed to verify that the explanation is being followed, and also usefully chunks the telling into shorter segments
- concludes the sequences with **new or repeated test questions** to verify that the trainee does indeed understand and/or to take the trainee's thinking or understanding further.

This explaining triad is a more effective teaching device than the pure didactic explanation alone, not least because it keeps the trainee actively participating rather than being a mere passive listener and it provides feedback to the trainer on whether the explanation is being understood.

Didactic talk provides the coach with very weak feedback on its impact on the trainee. A bored or puzzled trainee may reveal this state of mind through body language, but clever trainees learn to mask their boredom or incomprehension. If questions of whatever form are unanswered, this tells the coach something useful about the trainee. By contrast large quantities of didactic talk may wash over trainees without their betraying in any way their incomprehension or lack of interest.

ACTION POINTS ON TELLING AND EXPLAINING

- use test questions to verify trainees' current knowledge—it makes sure you don't cover ground unnecessarily
- 'chunk' telling by interspersing it with questions—don't just tell
- use regular check out questions to make sure that trainees are both listening and understanding
- learn how to use the explaining triad:
    - test questions (to uncover state of trainee knowledge)
    - explaining and check outs (to ensure trainee follows)
    - test questions (to verify trainee understands fully)
- try spells of thinking-out-loud or the running commentary to help trainees
- if you can successfully model thinking-out-loud and the running commentary, then encourage trainees to try it—but don't force it on them.

9 HOW TO GET AND GIVE FEEDBACK

Tra˙

> In my view, fair treatment of an individual means that he or she has every ɪ
> as closely as you can convey, what are the things that he or she can do better, ɑᴨɑ ᴡ…ᴜ–
> is the best course to take for the man or woman concerned in order to further their own
> interests.
>
> Sir John Harvey-Jones, industrialist, 1994

> All those involved in teaching can contribute by creating a positive educational
> environment, helping learners to achieve their goals by providing support and
> constructive feedback . . . They need to understand more about the need for, and
> ways of, achieving feedback, appraisal, openness and trust.
>
> The Report of SCOPME, 1994
> (The Standing Committee on Postgraduate Medical Education)

THIS SECTION:

- **illustrates the weakness of current feedback practices**
- **outlines the joint responsibilities of trainers and trainees**
- **illustrates good practices for both coach and trainee**
- **describes the dimensions of feedback**
- **explains the relationship between feedback and assessment**

Over a number of years, surveys have shown that lack of feedback is the most common complaint trainees make about their training. In many ways it is also the most serious, for feedback is essential to progression in learning. Bland reassurances are sometimes given, but this is not what trainees want.

TRAINEE COMMENTS ON FEEDBACK

He told me I was doing fine, that was it.

I don't feel I'm given enough information on where I stand.

What I'd like is more feedback directly from the Consultants on a day-to-day basis.

A lack of regular and clear feedback from the trainer condemns a trainee at best to learning by trial and error—hardly the best method. No wonder, then, that trainees enter a desperate search for external feedback beyond their self-evaluation.

63

..iees are driven to indirect sources:

- inferring that all is going well if the Consultant doesn't complain
- picking up 'vibes'; listening to hearsay about what the Consultant said
- making comparisons with one's peers
- guessing at one's competence on the basis of how well one is coping.

These are useful but not reliable guides.

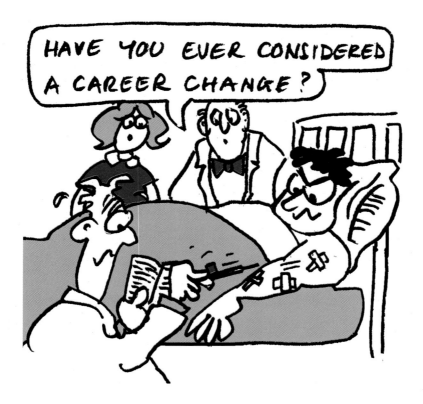

INDIRECT SOURCES OF FEEDBACK:TRAINEE REPORTS

You get feedback from Consultants either covertly or overtly. You do something, they're obviously very annoyed; you do something, they're obviously pleased. You learn to pick up the signals.

When the Consultant goes away, if he leaves you to do his outpatients' clinic, then you know you can be trusted.

> *The secretary's told me that one of the Consultants was quite impressed with me, but I haven't heard anything from the Consultant himself.*
>
> *I think the Consultants feel formal feedback might in some ways detract from the system, the apprenticeship system, the traditional system.*
>
> Unpublished 1994 Survey

Some trainees are reluctant to ask for direct feedback, for fear that it will be distressingly negative. Trainers are often embarrassed by the task and prefer to say as little as possible—though many seem to imagine that they give more and clearer feedback than their trainees believe. It is when both trainer and trainee back away from the task of giving and getting feedback that the trainee faces the greatest danger of progression in learning being inhibited.

> *It's very easy to be negative about feedback and think that no feedback is bad feedback. Short of somebody sitting you down and saying you're doing fine, you're not going to be happy with what you're doing. It's not easy to go and ask people saying: Am I alright? Nobody likes doing that because they're worried what the answer might be.*
>
> Trainee

We tend to think of feedback as a one-way communication, from trainer to trainee, and the responsibility for it as belonging to the trainer. This is a misconception. Feedback requires active work from both trainer and trainee.

> *I think traditionally the feedback junior doctors have got has been when things are going wrong and they've had their tails kicked. So if the opportunity arises when I hear that they've done something particularly well or a patient's been pleased or something, I think you need to take the opportunity to encourage them. I think that's useful. It's something that you've actually got to think about. I don't know how good many of us are at doing it. I think we need to create an environment where the juniors feel it's safe for them to lay themselves open to criticism in the knowledge that any criticism they will get will be constructive.*
>
> Trainer

We don't have any formal feedback. To the SHOs I try to be encouraging if I think they've done something well. There's no feedback structure. It's all very sensitive and you have to tread carefully. There is a lack of formal feedback in this department because no one wants to do it. There's a fair amount of drip feedback. The Consultant might say that one of the SHOs doesn't look happy or he's heard from Sister that he's been antagonising somebody, so will I have a word with him. There's that sort of paternalistic feedback to keep everybody on the straight and narrow. Or the Consultant says something good about an SHO, so I pass it on if I remember to keep morale up—everybody needs to know they're being appreciated. Personally, I would have welcomed somebody's appraisal of me. That would be valuable, because as you get more senior you don't know whether you're picking up totally bad habits and no one is going to tell you.

Specialist Registrar

You fill out a form assessing how you do in the various areas and your supervisor takes an average of all the Consultants' views and then you discuss it. I think it's helpful, but there's a certain kind of facelessness about it. You don't know which Consultant has said what and made which criticism. I don't find that particularly helpful because you end up with a series of marks and the median is just about average to good, which I suppose is what most of us expect. I find personal feedback more helpful. When I'm told on the job 'Good, you did that well today' or 'Yes, you showed some aptitude with that difficult case' that is very encouraging.

Trainee

The main responsibilities of the **trainer** in feedback are:

- to always be prepared to offer feedback
- to take the initiative in providing feedback
- to provide both positive feedback (e.g. what is being done well) and negative feedback (e.g. what is being done badly)
- to make the negative feedback highly specific and directed in a practical way to improvement, that is, it refers to concrete examples and is accompanied by advice or suggestion about how it can be done better in future.

The main responsibilities of the **trainee** in feedback are:

- always to be ready to receive feedback
- to take the initiative and ask for it if it is not offered
- to expect both positive and negative feedback

- to listen carefully to negative feedback, and to ask for some constructive, practical advice on how to remedy weaknesses or faults.

It is important that both coach and trainee treat the giving and the receiving of feedback as a crucial part of their relationship. For this reason they must do so from a very early stage in their relationship. If, sometimes with the best intentions, the trainer defers it for several weeks, then feedback becomes something the trainer would prefer to avoid and providing it is postponed yet again. As some trainees attest, it may then never be given at all. So trainees may have to ask for feedback. The trainee should give the coach some time to think about this.

A golden rule for trainees is this: if you don't get feedback, ask for it.

EXAMPLE OF A GOOD PRACTICE

Trainee to coach: *I've been working with you for 3 weeks now, and I suppose you're beginning to get an idea of how I'm doing. I appreciate that you've been giving me some space to settle into your firm, but I'm now ready to hear what you think of my work and get advice on how I might make progress. Could we arrange a time when we might have a short, informal chat about this later in the week?*

Thus the trainee takes the initiative in introducing feedback-giving into the training relationship but in a way that leaves the trainer feeling comfortable about providing it.

The coach remembers a very simple fact: most trainees are starved of feedback and want much more of it — but they do not feel they can say so to the trainer's face. A guide for trainers is this: praise in public but criticise in private. If trainers took the initiative and followed this simple precept, there would be a significant increase in trainee satisfaction with feedback.

Feedback touches on the most sensitive and emotional aspects of the relationship between trainer and trainee, and both are often alert to every nuance of their talk in this sphere. This is why many trainers are uncomfortable with it and often eschew

> ## EXAMPLE OF A GOOD PRACTICE
>
> Trainer to trainee: *You've been in the firm for a week or two now, and I hope you're beginning to settle in. Perhaps it would be a good idea if we had a short private chat about your progress later in the week. Nothing too formal, more a sharing of thoughts. I can give you my first impressions of how you're doing. I expect you'd like me to tell you where you're doing well, but we can also talk about where you want to make progress next. How about Tuesday after clinic?*

this responsibility. Giving clear indications of when milestones are passed and cushioning failure are not skills trainers feel confident they possess.

Yet for trainees such feedback touches upon their key concern about success or failure in the job and about whether they are making progress to the extent expected and at the proper rate.

So it is one thing to make sure that there are opportunities for feedback to be provided: it is another to make sure that the style and content of such feedback make the exercise constructive, worthwhile and supportive of trainee learning.

Feedback is easier and more supportive of learning if the **coach**:

- gives it reasonably close to the relevant trainee behaviour
- bases it wherever possible on what has been directly observed
- provides positive feedback as often as possible—most trainees are starved of it
- avoids indiscriminate or vague positive feedback and focuses on something specific
- where criticism is involved, criticises the trainee's behaviour, not the trainee as a person
- offers clear positive advice on what to do, not just on what not to do, in future.

and if the **trainee:**

- tries to avoid being defensive; trainees have generally been successful at school and university and find it hard after qualifying to find themselves making mistakes
- uses criticism as an occasion to seek detailed advice on how to get it right
- encourages the trainer to keep giving feedback—e.g. by saying 'thank you' for it—for the positive feedback will eventually come and be its own reward.

Feedback, then, is not a one-way process, but a commitment by both coach and trainee to co-operate in this most delicate but important aspect of training.

Feedback and assessment

Many trainers are more comfortable with providing formal, summative assessments after several months on the job, whereas trainees also want informal and frequent, formative feedback, integrated into OJT to guide their learning. Feedback and assessment are different but closely related concepts. They are often confused, so trainees are in danger of getting neither in any adequate form. Trainers and trainees need to clarify their thinking on the two concepts. The following set of antitheses helps.

THE DIMENSIONS OF FEEDBACK AND ASSESSMENT

Formal *versus* informal
An official or formal assessment *versus* an informal feedback not intended to have official standing.

Oral *versus* written
Feedback is usually spoken and rarely written, whereas assessment may be spoken but often is put in writing which may or may not be made available to the trainee.

Immediate *versus* delayed
Given during or directly after the performance of some action by a trainee *versus* postponed until some later stage. (Feedback may be immediate or delayed but assessment is normally delayed.)

69

Direct *versus* indirect
Provided personally by the coach to the trainee *versus* routed some other way—for example, a colleague reports to the trainee what the coach has said about him/her.

Positive *versus* negative
Praise or indication of approval *versus* criticism or indication of disapproval.

'Formative' *versus* 'summative'
Provided during a period of learning and intended to influence it *versus* provided as a terminal judgement at the end of a period of learning. (Feedback is formative more often than summative; assessment is more often summative than formative.)

Unilateral *versus* bilateral
Feedback and assessment from coach to trainee on quality of learning *versus* from trainee to coach on quality of teaching. (The unilateral approach is common. Where the coach introduces a bilateral element, the trainee is usually surprised and sometimes embarrassed.)

Trainees are looking for OJT feedback that is

- informal
- oral
- immediate
- direct
- formative
- unilateral from the trainer
- both positive and negative.

> *My dream for a training plan would be that every now and then a Consultant would come round and watch me doing my job and then afterwards say to me 'Now you should really have asked this question' or 'Why did you put your stethoscope there and not there?'*
>
> Trainee

> *My trainer sometimes says 'You've managed that very well. There's nothing for me to add.' That's very good. But that is a rare thing. Most of the feedback is negative, if you get it at all.*
>
> Trainee

The regular provision of such feedback is essential to the learning that leads to progression—and it is the foundation on which a later assessment (formal, written, delayed, summative) rests.

The feedback pyramid

The feedback pyramid consists of three layers, each being a different kind of feedback.

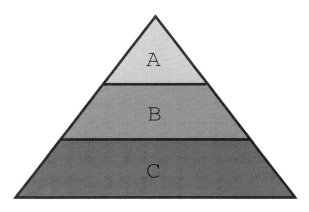

A = formal and summative feedback in an assessment.

There is a relatively small amount of this. If it occurs at all, it is provided by the coach in a rather formal way at the end of the period of training.

C = instant/short-term feedback on specific acts.

There is often a substantial amount of this form, both positive and negative, provided by the coach. The positive comes as the 'Well done' or 'That's good' and negative as 'No' or 'There's another way of doing that' when trainees are doing something wrong, inappropriate or dangerous.

B = holistic feedback on a sequence of acts.

It is this middle tier of the feedback pyramid—the feedback on a sequence of acts that belongs at the end of a coaching cycle—that so very often is missing and yet is a vital element in effective feedback.

One can't help but be aware of the fact that one of the trainees' most fundamental gripes is that they're not given enough feedback on how they are actually doing. They don't want to be told they're coping, they want to be told how they're doing. I try whenever possible to flag up good practice and say 'Well done' or 'That's good medicine' and I try, discreetly at the time, to say 'Well, I'm not sure I would have done that' or 'There are other ways of doing that' and 'Perhaps for this reason I might have chosen an alternative', knowing only too well one has to be very careful not to humiliate or insult the trainee in front of colleagues and patients because it destroys everyone's relationship with each other.

Trainer

Occasionally, cases come through on the ward and the outcome hasn't been what we might have hoped for. It's not necessarily anybody's fault, but we have a little informal post-mortem about if we'd done that, would it have worked out any different? There might be a medium-term discussion about things that would be regarded as thinking-training.

Trainer

A follow-up phase to a sequence of acts is the obvious way of providing the missing tier. This kind of holistic feedback makes a huge contribution to learning and progression in that in ideal terms it:

- allows the coach to give feedback on the trainee's behaviour in the episode as a whole
- allows the trainee to ask questions that might not have been possible or appropriate during service
- is retrospective in that it relates the feedback to the intentions made in the planning phase and also, if links are made with previous coaching cycles, potentially provides an evaluation of trainee progress
- is prospective in that it points forward to future learning needs and opportunities, thus feeding into later coaching cycles
- gives the coach an opportunity to offer advice/support.

This cannot be done all the time, of course. It needs, however, to be done regularly. OJT would be greatly improved if on some occasions trainee physicians were provided with feedback through an occasional follow-up session of a coaching cycle as the middle layer of the feedback pyramid.

Here are some suggestions to coaches on how to do it.

- following a service delivery session, such as a ward round, a clinic or a period on-take, the trainee is asked to review his/her performance
- following the treatment of a patient through the natural history of an illness, the trainee is asked to review the effectiveness of his/her management.

In both instances, coaches should:

- **Let the trainee start the review**

The trainee describes the good features of his/her performance/management. The coach may need to offer active encouragement here, since trainees are often unduly self-critical. The coach may need to add instances of what was done well.

- **Let the trainee examine what might have been done better**

The coach lets the trainee have the first shot at saying what he/she would have liked to do better or differently—and how and why. The coach then provides supportive advice through practical suggestions for improvement next time.

Sometimes the trainee may be unaware of weaknesses or deficiencies or unwilling to acknowledge them openly. This is the most delicate part of a feedback dialogue. Through careful questioning the coach leads the trainee both to analyse the nature and extent of the problem and to probe possible solutions to it. Trainees do not mind being told of their weaknesses if this is done in an objective, matter-of-fact way that does not come across as a personal attack. Again, the coach is positive in giving advice on where to find the relevant knowledge or how and where to acquire the relevant skill.

- **Enthuse the trainee**

Most trainees are anxious about how well they are doing and so may easily become disheartened. If trainees leave the feedback conversation feeling they have learnt something of worth and are looking forward to the occasion when they are confident their adjusted performance will be better, the coach can rest assured that the vital middle layer of the feedback pyramid is being provided.

- **Get feedback on your coaching skills**

Like any other learner, you need feedback if you want to get better at teaching, so ask the trainees for their views—be ready for some straight talking.

73

ACTION POINTS ON GIVING AND RECEIVING FEEDBACK

TRAINERS

- give lots of feedback—trainees need it to learn
- remember how much trainees are forced to rely on indirect feedback—which may give quite the wrong impression of your actual views
- offer both positive and negative feedback—constructively
- be specific with the feedback—avoid vague praise or blame
- praise in public; criticise in private
- criticise the behaviour, not the person
- ask for some feedback on your coaching—it will help you get better at it and your asking shows that you think feedback is essential to sound learning and improvement.

TRAINEES

- if you don't get much feedback, ask for some—be clear what you want and choose the moment when you ask for it.

TRAINERS AND TRAINEES

- learn the different types of feedback—give or ask for:
  —instant feedback on a specific act
  —holistic feedback on a sequence of acts (e.g. over a half-day)
  —formal, summative feedback at the end of training.

10 HOW TO IMPLEMENT A TRAINING PLAN

The physician develops more slowly than the surgeon and success comes later.
Sir William Osler, Regius Professor of Medicine,
University of Oxford, 1904

Set targets which are impossible to achieve and you switch people off. Set targets which are too easy and you also switch them off. Set targets which are difficult but just achievable, and then ensure that you achieve them, and you will switch people on.
Sir John Harvey-Jones, 1988

Educational supervisors can help by encouraging trainees to define their own educational objectives [and by] discussing and agreeing with trainees what should happen in order to meet these objectives, how this should be done, by whom, when and with what outcomes; in other words, to enter into an educational 'contract'.
The Report of SCOPME, 1994
(The Standing Committee on Postgraduate Medical Education)

THIS SECTION:
- **explains why a training plan is essential**
- **illustrates how to construct a training plan**
- **shows how to use a training plan to support the process of training**

Some trainees feel that they drift through their training; it is not the guided journey they expected at the beginning. Some trainees learn from bitter experience that training should be planned and that the initiative may lie with them.

I learned hardly anything on that job. One thing I did learn is that you should start each job with an objective. That's one thing I've lacked. It's a good thing to start a job with a list of the things that you want to get out of that 6 months or 3 months. Then when you see the job coming to an end, you can say to the Consultant: 'I haven't done this yet and my time with you is coming to an end, so d'you think I could learn to do this before my time's up?' If you start with a list of objectives you can keep track of what you're learning and it will give you a bit more direction in your training.
Trainee

Apprenticeship-by-coaching is structured training that is planned and monitored and then adjusted in the light of experience. Giving direction and purpose to training is a difficult ideal to achieve during clinical practice and service unless the coach and the trainee co-operate to agree upon a training plan to guide the process of training.

A training plan is an agreement between coach and trainee on what is to be achieved in a given period. It takes into account the trainee's previous experience, current levels of knowledge and skill, and aspirations for learning. It reflects the coach's pattern of work and the expectations of what the trainee can reasonably be expected to achieve.

What kind of training plan do coach and trainee want and need?

Every trainee is unique and comes to the attachment with a distinctive resource of experience, aptitudes and aspirations. The coach recognises that each trainee is hoping to gain from the attachment a unique combination of knowledge and skill which has somehow to be fitted into what the coach sees as an adequate and relevant training. The training agenda is thus a mix of what each party brings to the training.

A training plan works well if what the trainer considers to be the appropriate content of training can be adapted, by agreement, to the learning needs of a particular trainee. In other words, the ideal plan is not a rigid, bureaucratic one permitting no variations and imposed by the trainer on all trainees: rather it is a personalised plan which takes account of the trainee's learning needs and wishes as well as the trainer's expectations, requirements and resources. When coach and trainee have a hand in making such a plan, both have a stake in its success.

What is needed is a way of making each plan different but within a system that can achieve this quickly and efficiently without having to start from scratch with every trainee. The rest of this Section explains how this is done.

Designing a training plan

A training plan has four basic elements.

THE FOUR ELEMENTS OF A TRAINING PLAN

- List of topics to be covered during training

- Target for each topic

- Time-scale for achieving each target

- Record of targets achieved.

The **list of topics** to be covered is a mixture of knowledge and skills within the medical specialty concerned, determined to be relevant to the particular trainee for the specific training period.

An SHO expects to be involved in the assessment, diagnosis and management of the most common conditions within the specialty, but also expects to see more complex forms of common conditions as well as rarer conditions. Both trainee and coach also need to consider courses in preparation for examinations, and opportunities to learn about research. The precise character of the plan takes into account the variety of career aspirations or uncertainties found at SHO level.

In the case of a Specialist Registrar concentrating for a limited period on a sub-specialty, the topics may simply be a list of conditions to be assessed, diagnosed and managed.

The **target for each topic** is specified at an agreed level in a chosen scale of progression. An example of a scale of progression is given in the table on p. 18. The **time-scale for achieving each target** is usually straightforward — the training period. A more sophisticated way is to use the boxes to mark a time-frame — say, the first month for level 1, the second month for level 2, and the third month for level 3.

Before creating a plan for an individual trainee, the trainer has to do the general preparatory thinking to devise the base plan from which all individual plans will be derived. The trainer:

- sorts the conditions in the specialty by category of incidence — common, unusual or rare
- clarifies for each condition what constitutes simple and complex cases
- develops expectations about whether by the end of the training period, trainees at different levels of experience (an SHO's first job after registration, an SHO with 2 years' experience, Specialist Registrars with between 1 and 5 years experience in the specialty) should be able to deal with which conditions, with help or unaided.

Making a plan for a particular trainee

The trainer now:

- lists in the vertical column the conditions that this trainee might reasonably cover in some form during the period of training
- blanks out (or closes) all those boxes which are likely to be beyond the expected achievement of the trainee — for these will not be made into targets
- in the open boxes inserts some appropriate set of **ADM** initials.

A = trainee expected to assess the condition without help;   a = with help

D = trainee expected to diagnose the condition without help;   d = with help

M = trainee expected to manage the condition without help;   m = with help

This is illustrated in the two plans on pages 80 and 81, one for an SHO and one for a Specialist Registrar.

In some boxes the whole **ADM** set is relevant. In others, part of the set applies: for example, the trainee is expected to manage but not to diagnose.

Boxes are filled in across the horizontal axis, which specifies the setting to which the target applies. For some conditions the **ADM** set applies to all settings. For others, just one or two settings are appropriate. As an obvious example, some simple common conditions will be seen in out-patient clinics but not on the ward.

This kind of plan allows trainer and/or trainee to add idiosyncratic features. As examples:

- it may be useful to indicate the number of cases of a condition appropriate to a plan by putting a number in the box, since some conditions or procedures should be dealt with many times, whereas others perhaps just seen once
- some conditions may be assigned a particular priority in the trainee's learning and so be indicated by an asterisk (*)
- the trainer may want the trainee to learn to recognise some uncommon conditions very quickly (because, for instance, they are life-threatening) and these can be indicated by a dagger (†).

Both trainer and trainee now have a clear 'mental map' both of the specialty and of what the trainee is expected to achieve on that map. To implement the plan, the trainer and trainee take action to ensure that, wherever and whenever possible, the trainee is exposed to the right kinds of case at the right time.

Take the case of a new SHO, for whom both Consultant and Registrar will have a training role. In clinic, the trainee is immediately instructed in the whole ADM set for simple common conditions so that, if the trainer thinks it appropriate, he or she can contribute as soon as possible to service. Such cases are then filtered to the trainee, and the trainer moves on to instructing the trainee in complex versions of common conditions as well as simple versions of more unusual conditions, and so on. A similar planned progression is devised for other settings (wards, on-take etc.).

Though the two attached plans (Diagrams 2 and 3) look rather different, they follow the same basic principle. Indeed, they illustrate just how adaptable the scheme is, permitting considerable variation in the light of trainer and trainee needs and preferences.

A training plan for physicians.
Example: an SHO (general medicine)

CONDITION	Read	Tutorial	See	Assist	Do
				SETTING	
			CLINIC	WARD	ON-TAKE
COMMON					
Simple					
Urine infection			ADM	ADM	ADM
Gastroenteritis			ADM	ADM	ADM
Cellulitis			ADM	ADM	ADM
Pneumonia				ADM	ADM
Overdose					ADM
Deep vein thrombosis			ADM	ADM	ADM
Acute heart failure				ADM	ADM
Acute myocardial infarct			—	ADM	ADM
Complex					
Septicaemia			—	ADM	ADM
Intracranial bleed			—	AdM	AdM
Acute renal failure			—	AdM	AdM
Acute respiratory failure			—	AdM	AdM
UNUSUAL					
Simple					
Meningitis			—	ADM	ADM
Coeliac disease			ADM	ADM	—
Tuberculosis			AdM	AdM	AdM
Endocarditis			AdM	AdM	AdM
Complex					
Addison's disease			adm	adm	adm
Leukaemia			adm	adm	adm
Myxoedema coma			—	adm	adm
Vasculitis			—	—	—
RARE Unspecified		To be seen as they arise — no specific targets.			

PROCEDURES CONDITION	SUPERVISED	UNSUPERVISED
Simple		
Intravenous line	Y	Y
Urinary catheter	Y	Y
Nasogastric tube	Y	Y
Joint aspiration 1st	Y	
Joint aspiration 2nd		
Complex		
Chest drain 1st	Y	
Chest drain 2nd	Y	
Lumbar puncture 1st		
Lumbar puncture 2nd		
Central line 1st	Y	
Central line 2nd		
Pacing line 1st		
Pacing line 2nd		
Pacing line 3rd		

A training plan for physicians.
Example: a specialist registrar (year 3) (general medicine)

	Read	Tutorial	See	Assist	Do
				SETTING	
CONDITION			CLINIC	WARD	ON-TAKE
UNUSUAL					
Simple					
Sarcoidosis			ADM	ADM	—
Wilson's disease			ADM	ADM	—
Cerebral malaria			ADM	ADM	ADM
Diabetes insipidus			ADM	ADM	
WPW			ADM	ADM	ADM
Complex					
HOCM			ADM	ADM	
AIDS			ADM	ADM	
SLE			AdM	ADM	
Amyloidosis			AdM	AdM	
Multiple endocrine neoplasia			AdM	AdM	
RARE					
Simple					
Benign intracranial hypertension			ADM	ADM	ADM
Haemachromatosis			ADM	ADM	—
Pituitary adenoma			ADM	ADM	ADM
Thyroid crisis			AdM	AdM	ADM
Syphilis			AdM	AdM	
Zollinger–Ellison			AdM	AdM	
Myasthenic crisis			AdM	AdM	ADM
Complex					
Goodpastures			AdM	AdM	
Dermatomyositis			adm	AdM	
Histiocytosis			adm	AdM	
Alveolar proteinosis			adm	AdM	
Löffler's syndrome			adm	adm	
Pearson's syndrome			adm	adm	
Gerstmann–Sträussler–Scheinker syndrome			adm	adm	—

Using the training plan

The training plan is just a document — a mere piece of paper — unless it is used as a tool to give direction and coherence to the training process. The plan is held by the trainee who keeps it handy throughout the attachment. As a target is reached, this is checked on the plan. The trainee takes responsibility for monitoring progression and takes action to steer training to those aspects of the plan that are in danger of

81

being neglected or overlooked. For example, the trainee may remind the coach from time to time about progress (or lack of it) being made or may take action to ensure that he/she gets access to those conditions and/or settings which are not being covered at the expected rate.

A conscientious coach may ask to look at the plan from time to time, partly to monitor progression and partly to remind him/herself of what remains to be done.

A joint look at the plan is particularly useful when discussing a forthcoming ward round or clinic, so that the targets can influence the role the trainee is to adopt in relevant procedures or cases as a kind of training 'menu' for that occasion.

In this way the balance of training swings away from the opportunistic and unplanned to planned and progressive OJT with minimal intrusion into service provision.

A training plan also makes it easier for coach and trainee to talk about training. Short meetings linked to the plan provide continuity and progression throughout the training period. Coach and trainee naturally talk informally about both training and service as part of their daily work, but ideally coach and trainee need to meet rather more formally, in protected time, to construct the plan; to monitor progress; and then to evaluate whether the plan has been realised. Trainers and trainees normally have a meeting at the beginning and end of the attachment. This Section advises on how these meetings can, with the clearer structure provided by the plan, be of greater value to coach and trainee.

Training meetings

We suggest two key training meetings, each lasting about 20 minutes, one at the beginning of the attachment to create the plan, and one at the end of the attachment to evaluate it. Both meetings are held by the coach in a quiet place in protected time for both. This takes effort on both sides, but the benefits are considerable.

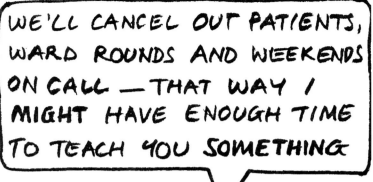

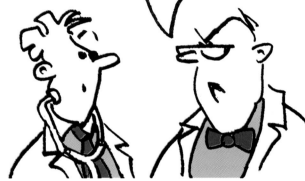

The planning meeting

> ### AGENDA FOR THE PLANNING MEETING
>
> Trainee's background, experience, aspirations
> Firm/team/department timetable
> Trainee's responsibilities
> Negotiation of a personalised plan

This is held as soon as possible after the trainee's arrival. Coach and trainee introduce themselves to 'break the ice'. The coach takes care to set the trainee at ease — he/she may well be apprehensive — since an honest and open relationship is a prerequisite for good training.

83

The coach has the following initial agenda:

- ask the trainee to describe previous posts and experience (and so bring a CV to the meeting)
- ask the trainee about their career hopes, intentions and plans
- ask the trainee about their examination record and intentions
- ask the trainee about recent and relevant clinical experience.

This gets the trainee making an early and active contribution to the discussion and demonstrates the coach's interest in the trainee. In the second part of the agenda the coach talks about:

- the service commitment of the job e.g. ward work, out-patients, on-call etc.
- the weekly timetable of work, including free time/study time
- what is expected of the trainee (in-patients, out-patients, on-call, other)
- the people in the firm/team and department with whom the trainee will be working, including their routines and styles.

In the last part of the initial meeting, the coach describes the partnership aspect to the training and encourages the trainee to take an active responsibility for his/her own training. The concept of OJT and its relation to service delivery is explained.

It is easiest to explain the training plan by showing the trainee a draft copy, based on the experience of similar previous trainees. An experienced trainee will be able to proceed to negotiating the plan there and then. The coach and trainee discuss, negotiate and complete the plan. It is important at this stage to stress that the plan is not a standard document but is to be personalised through discussion. Modification, perhaps extensive, is the norm. The trainee may suggest changes to the topics and target steps, and which boxes should be opened and closed. This is the first opportunity for the trainee to be pro-active and for the coach to show flexibility and responsiveness.

Less experienced trainees, and those new to the hospital and/or specialty, may be too overloaded with new information to contribute properly. Such trainees take the plan away for reflection and come to a further meeting a few days later to devise the plan in detail.

Once the plan has been agreed, the coach arranges for the final version to be typed up and returned to the trainee. If a master copy is kept on a computer, the personalised version can be produced easily and quickly.

It is essential that coach and trainee monitor the plan during the training period. From time to time either should take the initiative, in a free moment or over coffee, to check on progress. Some may prefer to have a short meeting of a rather more formal kind around the middle of the attachment.

A **mid-term discussion** provides the opportunity for coach and trainee to:

- examine the extent to which the agreed plan has been executed
- check the extent of the trainee's progress in reaching the targets
- record where targets have been reached or exceeded
- analyse the reasons if any aspects of the plan have fallen short
- revise or modify the plan/add or change topics
- identify key topics or targets on which training should focus.

Where logistical or learning problems emerge, coach and trainee agree strategies to ensure that they are overcome within a modified plan. For example, some conditions listed in the plan may never have been seen at all; or it had been planned that the trainee be exposed to a particular number of cases of a common condition, but in fact only one or two have been seen; or the trainee has learned how to diagnose a condition but has not yet been involved in its management. The mid-term discussion allows for corrective action to be drawn up.

The evaluation meeting

AGENDA FOR THE EVALUATION MEETING

Review the plan
Offer summative assessment
Link to next attachment
Get feedback on coaching

85

This is held towards the end of the post to conclude the training agreement and evaluate the effectiveness of the training plan and the achievements of the trainee.

This meeting will be of great significance to the trainee, since this is the occasion where the coach provides the summative feedback which serves as the formal assessment of trainee progress through the whole period of the attachment. There is positive feedback on the trainee's specific achievements in relation to the milestones of the specialty. New targets are outlined. In areas of relative weakness, the coach explores strategies for improvement which may well be carried forward into the next attachment.

It is not, however, just a one-way process, for the coach invites the trainee to comment on the quality of training. If the relationship is open and positive, neither party need be embarrassed. Comments on those areas where the training has been particularly supportive, as well as on areas where more help might have been useful, make this meeting reciprocally valuable. The coach cannot expect to get better at coaching in the absence of a judicious mix of detailed positive and negative feedback from trainees.

ACTION POINTS ON DESIGNING AND
IMPLEMENTING A TRAINING PLAN

TRAINERS

- make time for the meetings — it's worth the effort

- the first and last meetings (the welcome/planning and farewell/ feedback) are the most important — your trainee takes them as an index of how much you value both training and the trainee

- the agenda for the **initial meeting**
  - trainee background, experience, aspirations
  - firm/team/department timetable
  - trainee's responsibilities
  - negotiation of a personalised training plan

- the agenda for the **final meeting**
  - review the plan
  - offer summative assessment
  - link to the next attachment
  - get feedback on your coaching

- during the attachment, keep referring to the plan to steer and modify OJT — mid-course corrections are usually necessary

- encourage the trainee to record progression through OJT

- don't make the document (the plan) more important than the process of planning.

87

11 OJT ON THE WARD

Sir Lancelot strode across the ward, drew up sharply, and looked over the patients in the two rows of beds, sniffing the air like a dog picking up a scent. He thundered over to the bedside of a small, nervous man in the corner. The firm immediately rearranged itself, like a smart platoon at drill. The Chief towered on the right of the patient's head; Sister stood opposite, her nurses squeezed behind her; the students surrounded the foot and sides of the bed like a screen; and the Registrar and houseman stood beyond them, at a distance indicating that they were no longer in need of any instruction in surgery.

Richard Gordon, medical humorist, 1952

The physician needs a clear head and a kind heart; his work is arduous and complex, requiring the exercise of the very highest faculties of the mind, while constantly appealing to the emotions and finer feelings.

Sir William Osler, Regius Professor of Medicine,
University of Oxford, 1904

THIS SECTION:

- **describes the wide variations in ward round practices and structures**
- **shows how to implement a coaching cycle on ward rounds**
- **describes four types of ward rounds**
- **relates the four types of ward rounds to the achievement of training goals**
- **explains the 3-minute round-up and the case presentation progression.**

The teaching ward round is a hallowed tradition of the teaching hospital and images of it — not least James Robertson Justice as Sir Lancelot Spratt — are locked in the collective memory of all doctors, physicians and surgeons alike.

The teaching ward round is, however, just one type of round. Others include: business rounds, Consultant-led rounds, rounds led by a Specialist Registrar/Senior House Officer, on-take rounds and post-take rounds. All types are potentially rich in opportunities for fusional OJT.

The common practice of distinguishing between a business ward round and a teaching ward round may be unhelpful, for it implies that some rounds are, and should be, teaching free. This is neither true, for there will be teaching and learning

89

on any ward round, nor desirable, for the art of fusional OJT is blending teaching and learning into service. In other words, all ward rounds, whatever their designated purpose, whether they are formal or informal, long or short, should be treated as occasions when teaching and learning could and should take place. There is a broad spectrum, with at one extreme some having relatively little explicit teaching and learning, and at the other extreme some containing a substantial amount of training, some of which has been carefully planned and/or followed up.

So, both coach and trainee treat every ward round as a training opportunity. The post-take round is particularly useful because of the follow-up of patients seen by the firm. Rounds relatively free of time constraints are obviously ideal for training, since this gives the coach more time for OJT that may be somewhat intrusive upon service delivery — for example, to encourage the trainee to ask questions and to allow the trainee to deliver part of the service. A long ward round in a limited time reduces the time for teaching, but does not remove it entirely, provided the coach is skilled in fusional OJT.

Define roles, responsibilities and aims of ward rounds

Learning how to assess, diagnose, investigate and manage are central to the trainee physician's aspirations. So the provision of real opportunities for this by the coach is of paramount importance. Trainee physicians who feel that they are peripheral to the decision-making processes on wards will be dissatisfied by their training and may show signs of low morale.

Effective OJT requires that the coach finds, for each trainee, the most appropriate balance between giving them enough responsibility, and providing them with adequate supervision and support.

> *Trainees do want to have a certain amount of stretching, they do want a certain amount of responsibility, but they want frequently to be able to 'check in' with their Consultants just to say 'I've done this, is everything all right?' Even the more senior know that the feeling of support is very important.*
> Trainer

Finding the most appropriate balance of responsibility and support is an important task for the coach. The courageous Consultant is willing to ask these three key questions of juniors:

- are you being given enough responsibility?
- are you being stretched?
- are you being adequately supervised and supported?

If the answer is 'no' to any of these, then rectifying action is vital.

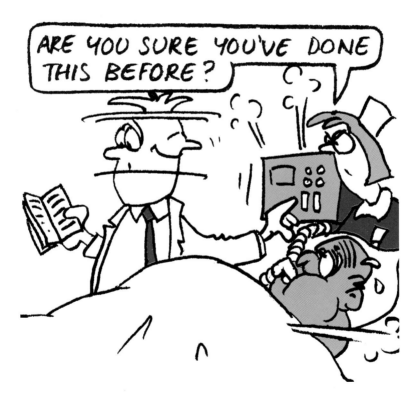

The sliding scale of ward rounds, from those with little explicit teaching and learning, to those with a substantial amount of training, implies an explicit understanding of the aims and objectives of the various types. In practice, few trainers and trainees share such an understanding.

91

> *Perhaps the expectation of all of us was rather different in terms of what we were aiming to do. It's quite clear that the trainees' expectations of what is available in terms of teaching, training and learning on a ward round is different from mine.*
>
> Trainer

Where individual enthusiasm does not drive the teaching, there is a danger that the teaching element gets squeezed out and rounds become focused exclusively on service. In the absence of clear training aims and expectations, the teaching element may be difficult to sustain across all types of round. Fusional OJT requires trainers and trainees to share an explicit understanding of ward round aims and expectations and the place of teaching and learning within them.

> *The teaching and learning process was inhibited by people not knowing the objectives of the ward round and it would be very wise to establish the objectives of the ward rounds early on. One could sit down sometime at the beginning of the attachment and just have one session on what is the purpose of the ward round and so establish a structure of the ward round and what takes place when. We ought to make it quite clear that this is going to be the routine and that this is going to happen.*
>
> Trainer
>
> *I tell them what they can expect of me and what I expect of them on the ward round.*
>
> Trainer

Coaches ask themselves:

- what are the aims of each ward round and where do teaching and learning fit into them?
- can opportunities for teaching and learning be maximised by making selective aspects an agreed priority on specified rounds?
- how can ward rounds be arranged and administered so that teaching and learning do not get 'squeezed out' by service demands?

Develop OJT skills and practices

Ward rounds offer many opportunities for a wide range of teaching techniques — modelling, demonstrating, explaining, asking questions — over many basic topics, clinical, administrative and generic.

Clinical:

- history (presentation patterns, eliciting important symptoms clearly)
- examination (eliciting physical signs)
- assessment and diagnosis
- planning and interpretation of investigations
- patient management (explanation, counselling)
- instructions for ward staff
- treatment planning
- treatment monitoring, detection of complications
- planning rehabilitation.

Administrative:

- dealing with relatives
- consent
- support services (social and community)
- discharge
- management of the firm/team and other professional colleagues.

Generic communication and social skills may be modelled, taught and practised, including the following:

- establishing rapport with patients
- developing the art of listening
- obtaining accurate information in history taking
- eliciting fears and anxieties (declared or undeclared)
- interpreting non-verbal behaviour (e.g. facial expression, body position)
- using appropriate non-verbal behaviour (e.g. seating position)
- responding to concerns and worries
- explaining investigations and procedures
- explaining a diagnosis and its implications
- discussing treatment options
- breaking bad news
- checking that one is being understood.

The importance of the different teaching techniques will vary according to the type of round being conducted and the trainee's learning needs. For example,

93

feedback is particularly relevant for the trainee on a post-take ward round and explanation will be central where the trainee has only a basic knowledge of the case or condition concerned.

Remember that trainees may be reluctant to ask questions in front of patients if they think that asking a question will undermine the confidence that patients have and need in their competence. For the same reason, they may not be responsive to questions from the coach if an answer is likely to expose their ignorance, or even worse, errors of some kind. From the trainee's point of view, questions on a ward round always carry the risk of leading to public humiliation. The effective coach develops strategies of asking questions in a way which does not threaten the patient or learner, or develops a practice of encouraging trainees to save up questions until after the ward round.

Examine the teaching potential of every ward round

Ward rounds potentially have a structure parallel to that of the coaching cycle.

PHASES OF A COACHING CYCLE

Planning phase where coach and trainee decide the aspect of training on which to focus

Service delivery phase into which OJT is fused or blended

Follow-up phase where coach and trainee review the quality of trainee performance and any training provided and decide what to do in the next training cycle.

PHASES OF A WARD ROUND

Before the ward round = **planning phase**

The ward round itself = **service delivery phase with OJT**

After the ward round = **follow-up phase**

As with coaching cycles, all three phases of the ward round are rarely undertaken on any one occasion. The important issue is that the functions of each phase are covered in some form at some time during the period of training.

Let us consider each in turn.

Before the ward round — a planning phase (for both training and service delivery)

> I think that a long, disorganised, standing up, overcrowded ward round is the worst possible teaching setting. Sitting in a comfortable, pleasant, airy room for a discussion before the round in a relaxed atmosphere is very conducive.
>
> Trainee
>
> What would be useful on a ward round would be if you went through a list of the patients before you actually went round. It's much better to talk about a patient before seeing them. I once had a trainer who said 'The best ward rounds are those you do without notes.' Then you don't speak about the patient but to the patient.
>
> Trainee

Planning training opportunities is part of good coaching. However, the degree to which opportunities can be planned is highly dependent upon the level of advance knowledge about patients held by the trainer and/or the trainee(s). Where at least one team member is familiar with the patients to be seen, there is considerable scope for planning the teaching opportunities.

This planning phase — seen by many trainees as the key to ward round training — is best done in an office or side-room on the ward. The trainee presents the Consultant and the others present (other junior doctors, nurses, paramedical staff) with an update on each patient in turn. The coach may offer explanations and ask questions of trainees and then give them an opportunity to ask questions.

Both coach and trainee review the patient list for training opportunities, which will constantly vary. It is possible to select from the list of patients a small number for special attention as a focus for teaching and learning because they relate to the trainee's training plan or learning needs at this time. This can be regarded as 'the training menu for the day'. The aim is to reach an agreement on three things:

95

- which patients/conditions are purely or largely service delivery
- which patients/conditions have significant opportunities for training
- which patients/conditions should make the round's 'training menu for the day', that is, the ones which, in relation to the training plan, are to be the focus for teaching and learning.

The coach obviously takes the lead here, but the trainee sometimes needs to take the initiative in promoting the review itself or in negotiating the training menu. This includes reminding the coach of the level the trainee has reached and aspires to with each condition.

The fact that the patient is not present allows:

- a full and frank discussion of the differential diagnosis and an assessment of the patient's condition and circumstances, including personality and character as it affects management
- questioning by the coach, with the trainees being able to offer answers in private without embarrassment
- open correction by the coach of unwise or erroneous answers and suggestions from trainees
- a debate on the advantages and disadvantages of various management and assessment options
- an analysis of the degree of success of a treatment and its effects and consequences
- a comparison by the Consultant with other similar cases, either currently on the ward or from the past
- a decision on the next steps in the management of the patient, after discussion of all the options and their merits
- a discussion on what needs to be done in relation to each patient on the ward round itself
- a selection of particular cases or patients or topics that make the 'training menu of the day'.

Each of these is an opportunity for teaching and learning.

The Consultant does not always have to be present during the planning phase: the trainees can prepare a training menu for a ward round before the coach arrives.

96

The ward round — (mainly) service delivery phase

If there has been a planning phase, the round itself may be relatively short. Much of the time will be taken up in reaffirming the relationship between patient and Consultant (and other members of the firm) — offering reassurance, boosting confidence and morale, providing information and checking that the patient has no outstanding problems, questions or complaints.

Any action decided in the planning phase — such as a physical examination — flows naturally. Other topics on the training menu, such as communication skills, can be modelled by the trainer or undertaken by the trainee. Some aspects of training are best achieved if the trainee leads the round, with the trainer supporting, advising and debriefing at the end.

> *I try and give the SHO the lead for part of the round so that I can see if they're getting competent and they're getting the confidence to lead. It immediately identifies where their weaknesses are and whether they can make sense of it all.*
>
> Trainer

If there has been no planning phase, the coach needs to be alert to the danger that the business aspect of the round will squeeze out the training aspect.

Being alert to unexpected opportunities for teaching is also part of good coaching. As the firm moves between patients the coach makes any additional comments and trainees ask questions that spring to mind from bedside observation. Issues are addressed as they arise, avoiding the danger of being lost.

> *In certain circumstances, you are taking a fuller history, you're doing things in more detail in the hope that the trainees will pick that up, but if they don't realise that's what you're doing, then they go off and do something different. And I don't know how to get over that because I don't want to say 'Now look, I'm doing a little teaching session here for you, what about it?' Somewhere you'd like to say 'Look, I'm really trying not only for me, but also for you to observe.' It's very difficult for a Consultant or for the trainer in that sort of working environment to say 'Look I'm now switching into training mode.' I'd like to have some sort of light that goes up — a signal to the trainee to listen in here because I'm trying to make a point!*
>
> Trainer

When trainers do find many opportunities for inserting training into service, they must make sure that trainees are alert enough not to miss them.

After the ward round — (mainly training) follow-up phase

The firm retires to an office or side-room, preferably where there is comfortable seating and refreshments. The team then discuss the issues arising from the ward round.

> *I try and end the ward round with a coffee — that's the time when the working part of the round is finished — and I think of what we've seen on the ward round.*
>
> Trainer

If there has been a planning phase, this final session will tend to be short, as the business is mainly a matter of confirming the soundness of decisions drafted in the planning phase or changing them in the light of evidence emerging during the round.

If there has been no planning phase, the session may well be longer, as there is an opportunity to engage in discussion of the topics and issues noted above. In such a discussion it is essential that trainees are encouraged to identify topics and issues, to ensure that their learning needs are addressed.

The follow-up session should also provide feedback (see Section 9). It does not matter if this is very short indeed, but trainees always want to know how well they have performed, particularly on post-take ward rounds where they have been responsible for the patient until someone more senior advises them. Simple praise is always welcome, provided that it is not done by formula and on appropriate occasions is supplemented by a more detailed talking through of what went well and what might have been done differently and in what way. Progression depends on a few moments of effective feedback.

Types of ward round and their teaching potential

In spite of the usual distinction between teaching and business ward rounds, it is fruitful to see ward rounds as being of four types.

TYPES OF WARD ROUND

Type 1 — ward round only
Type 2 — planning phase and ward round
Type 3 — ward round and follow-up phase
Type 4 — planning phase and ward round and follow-up phase.

Type 1 is very common but has the least teaching potential. Only where rounds of this type are very carefully managed will the learning opportunities presented successfully meet the learning needs of trainees.

Types 2 and 3 strike a good balance between the need to use time efficiently and the need to use the ward round as a vehicle for training.

Some trainers use either type 2 or type 3 as standard, but each has different strengths and using them in combination is both possible and beneficial. Type 2 is particularly useful when the trainees are new and/or relatively inexperienced, since the open discussion before the round supports rapid learning. Type 3 is useful as trainees acquire more experience and familiarity with the specialty and with the Consultant — and of course it is type 3 which is useful when time is pressing, since the follow-up can, under pressure, be brief.

Type 4 is very rare but has the richest teaching potential.

With discipline and a good organisation/planning of rounds, type 4 could be the rule rather than the exception.

Trainee

Two techniques to develop OJT

The 3-minute round-up

Every ward round should, at its conclusion, offer trainees a chance to put questions to the coach. Even the busiest trainer can afford to offer trainees the 3-minute round-up.

99

> If, at the end of the ward round, there is no follow-up phase, then the coach can say to the trainee(s):
>
> *The next 3 minutes are exclusively yours. You will have my full attention and nothing will interrupt us. Ask me anything at all, either arising from the ward round or because there is something since we last met that you want to talk about. OK, fire away.*

We guarantee that trainers will find that trainees do have questions to ask and points to make: the 3 minutes will be used up. Of course, the coach may be able to give more than 3 minutes; what is important is that the time period is clear and that it is dedicated exclusively to the trainee's questions and comments. Where the time period expires, the coach is free to say that time is up, and further questions must be banked until the next session.

The value of the 3-minute round-up is that:

- it ensures a teaching element in every ward round, even type 1
- it reaffirms to trainees that the coach is taking teaching as a priority
- it gives trainees some 'sacred' space which they value greatly
- it encourages trainees to store up good questions both from the ward round and from elsewhere, and makes sure they are answered before (as is too often their fate) they are forgotten.

Here is a trainer's opinion of the 3-minute round-up:

> *It's a way of bringing some sort of organisation to the ward round in our department. In my experience, it's often chaotic because 30% of the patients certainly I, and sometimes both my juniors, have not seen before, so one can't plan the ward round beforehand; there are too many imponderables. It's busy with lots of time pressures on us, so we can't have half-hour sessions discussing in-depth things, but it gives an opportunity that we all know is there if we need it. And it's manageable. Even if you've got something to do next, if you arrive 3 minutes late, no-one's going to turn a hair, so to have something on a scale which is actually manageable, and practicable, is important. And it actually is a way of empowering trainees, putting the ball in their court and letting them set the agenda for their needs and it shows them that you want to encourage them to be involved in the process.*

Use case presentations to aid progression in learning

In many specialties case presentation is an integral part of the ward round. The way that cases are presented will change in line with trainee's developing knowledge and experience.

Presentations usually cover three levels:

- the facts of the case
- the analysis of the facts
- the next steps and action points.

Over time trainees are helped by the coach to progress from determining the relevant facts, through the analysis of them, to finally making the decisions. Taking account of the pressure on time, and the trainee's experience and confidence, the coach moves the trainee along the graduated steps from contributing at the first level only to 'running the whole show'.

A trainee may be able to conduct the whole presentation for a reasonably straightforward case, whilst being at the first level for rare or complex conditions.

ACTION POINTS ON OJT ON THE WARD

TRAINERS

- treat every ward round, in some ways and at some parts, as a teaching round, especially if you have some that are designated teaching rounds

- on each ward round select the model most appropriate to the trainees' needs and the circumstances/pressures prevailing at the time:

  > Model 1 — ward round only (designated teaching
  >   or business)
  > Model 2 — planning phase and ward round
  > Model 3 — ward round and follow-up phase
  > Model 4 — planning phase and ward round and
  >   follow-up phase

- make sure everybody involved understands why you vary ward round models and don't use the same one every time

- in the planning phase, work out a training menu for the trainee(s) or encourage them to devise one of their own to focus their learning

- use the 3-minute round-up every time and encourage trainees to remind you about it in case you forget

- use case presentations to aid progression in learning

- let trainees conduct some ward rounds — but remember that they'll feel discouraged if, without giving reasons, you take over part way through.

12 OJT IN CLINIC

> In the eighteenth century, there were only teaching clinics... The clinic was concerned only with the instruction...that is given by a master to his pupils.
>
> Michel Foucault, philosopher, 1963
>
> The guiding principle of education in the clinic must be that of flexibility.
>
> Donald A West & Arthur Kaufman, medical educators, 1981

THIS SECTION:

- **describes five models of training in clinics**
- **shows how the models apply at different stages in training**
- **advises on how to get the best training out of clinic**

In recent years the move towards more out-patient care and less in-patient care has made the clinic setting an important and, some physicians argue, an under-utilised component of junior doctors' training. Pressures of time and patient numbers result in busy clinics heavily oriented to service delivery, but this does not remove all opportunities for OJT.

Clearly there could be better training if there were fewer patients or more Consultants. Better training may also be achieved through improved techniques of teaching and learning in clinic and the planning of training that is structured.

Organising the clinic for learning

There are very many ways of organising a clinic; Consultants, nurses and managers all have preferred ways.

For the clinic to run efficiently, three problems have to be solved:

- the filtering of patients to doctors: which patient sees which doctor — SHO, Specialist Registrar, Consultant
- the achievement of a reasonable through-put (especially if the clinic is busy) and of reasonable waiting times for patients
- the insertion of training into the above structure of service.

103

If they are to maximise the teaching opportunities, trainers must consider the following issues:

- the trainee's learning needs, as identified by their training plan, their experience and level of progression and the role and responsibilities they are equipped to take on
- how patients can be filtered to trainees to ensure that their learning needs are addressed and a reasonable patient through-put is achieved
- the level and organisation of support and supervision required by trainees.

Decisions about filtering of cases and the organisation of supervision may well be influenced by the extent to which the trainer is prepared to delegate patient management decisions. Maximising training opportunities at the minimal cost of intruding into service delivery is achieved when Consultant and trainee commit themselves to a kind of contract in which the trainer agrees to be generous in giving away opportunities to take the lead in seeing patients and the trainee in return demonstrates trustworthiness by seeking help whenever necessary.

The giving away element in the contract occurs when Consultants are willing to give away to their trainees as much clinical experience as they can, consistent with patient care and through-put.

The seeking help element in the contract occurs when trainees, conscious that they are being given clinical experience close to the limit of their knowledge and skill, must be ready to seek advice, help and intervention when it is needed and not wait for the Consultant to initiate it. But this will not happen unless Consultants take the lead in encouraging trainees to seek help — and trainees believe that the Consultants expect to be taken at their word.

> I'm not going to sit on your shoulder like a parrot for your time with me, because that put me off when I was in training. But I am always going to be available and I'll come to you at the drop of a hat. What I want you to do is tell me when you're not happy and then I'll come and do it for you if necessary. I'm going to assume that no communication from you means you are happy in your part of the clinic.
>
> Trainer to Trainee

> I like the amount of clinics that I do because that's a good way to learn. You have enough autonomy to do your own thing and to learn and to get involved, but there's always somebody there if and when you need them. You're never in a position where you feel 'I can't ask' when things are starting to go wrong. That's important. Part of the learning process is that you need time on your own but you must never be in a position where you feel there's no back-up. It's not easy for the trainer to get the balance right.
>
> Trainee

The contract between trainer and trainee means that the trainer gives away generously but on the understanding that the trainee will not waste time and pretend to non-existent understanding but will immediately call for advice, help or intervention when it is needed. Coach and trainee make a contract of trust. The trainee trusts that clinical experience will be forthcoming; the coach trusts the trainee to ask for help; the trainee trusts that this will not cause a reduction in the amount of clinical experience the coach will offer in future.

> If you have a problem, you ask for help. If the bosses are approachable, then you get trained without having formal teaching sessions once a week. I can remember an SHO whose problem was that he didn't ask for help. In the end somebody had to see all his patients in clinic, because he was dangerous. He had to be supervised all the time and so didn't get the normal learning by experience under supervision. All that sort of trainee can do is fill out the forms. So juniors are heavily supervised in clinic until you get to know them.
>
> Trainer

What are the main models of how clinics function and how training is fitted into the *modus operandi*? Of the many ways of organising them, five are selected as working models of the clinic.

Model 1 — sitting in

Here the trainer gets on with service delivery whilst the trainee observes. Whilst dealing with patients, the coach demonstrates, explains and asks questions of the trainee. In addition, the trainee may be sent from the consulting room or left in an examination room to deal with an aspect of management that is within his/her competence, subsequently resuming observation of the coach.

> *When I was a trainee, I'd been doing [this specialty] for quite some time when I actually sat in a clinic with one of my Consultants and watched her at work. It was a very different learning experience. I was surprised at how much I learnt. It was often more to do with how to talk to people, how to manage them, how to respond to them—all the good things to say and how to explain to patients. A surgical trainee would watch their boss operate. You can't become a physician just by watching, but that doesn't mean that you can't learn some important things by sitting in clinic and watching.*
>
> Consultant
>
> *Some out-patients are very stressed, and sometimes their worst qualities come out— we've got long waiting times in clinic and people get cross. So you do have to face people who are very difficult or very aggressive, and it can be quite unpleasant. I've definitely calmed down in my approach to people. I hold my ground and try to explain things properly but I never argue back. I've watched [one Consultant] in clinic and he is completely unruffleable, even with the most psychotic person. He does not rise to difficult people and I watch him and learn from that.*
>
> Trainee

Advantages are:

- trainees may receive a reasonable amount of training
- trainees see the full range of cases, including the rare or unusual, not just a filtered selection.

Disadvantages are:

- the trainee may lose concentration or get bored by just watching
- limited hands-on experience for the trainee
- the OJT is intrusive into service, so with just one doctor engaged in service the through-put of patients is slowed

- some trainers cannot afford this model because clinics are too busy, so coaching deteriorates to osmosis.

TRAINER AND TRAINEE DEBATE CLINIC MODELS

Trainee: *The way it was organised in clinic, I was supposed to sit in at the beginning and then do clinics on my own and if I had a question, I could ask the Consultant. I would have liked sitting in followed by reverse sitting in—I watch the Consultant do his clinic and then he watches me do mine. That way I would have learnt very quickly how to do the clinic correctly. I wish that could be done in all medical training. It could be better, it could be optimal because, by not doing it that way, the trainee makes many small mistakes which have no great consequences which take the Consultant's time at some different point.*

Trainer: *I've never thought about reverse sitting in before. The concern I have is the psycho-dynamics of the interview. The patient might realise that there's a Consultant in the corner and that might affect the relationship with the doctor in the chair. That's not necessarily insurmountable. I could say to patients, 'I shall be here, but I want my SHO to do the interview' and so actively engage the patient in the process. The main problem, of course, is the time component—if I'm watching you, I don't have time to see my own patients.*

Trainee: *Yes, I see that in the short term, but it might save time eventually, because if I don't get confidence quickly and learn what to do, then I just store up problems for somebody else further down the line, which takes up time.*

Model 2 — service-led training

Here trainees see patients directly as a contribution to service. Patients may be filtered so that trainees see only new patients, or only follow-up patients, or they may see any patient depending on their turn. Trainees deal with patients within their competence until they need advice, when they interrupt service delivery to check up the line. The coach may also interrupt service, for example, to invite the trainee to see an interesting or relevant case.

Advantages are:

- a high through-put of patients, since all doctors are engaged in service
- minor cases can be dealt with by trainees, to whom they may routinely be filtered.

Disadvantages are:

- a trainee may be excessively reluctant to seek advice from a coach, resulting in sub-standard service
- the trainee postpones the real decision, e.g. tells the patient to make another appointment in 3 months time
- training is unplanned and in danger of containing an unstructured or random selection of cases
- trainees easily become restricted to simple or straightforward cases and their progression is thus limited
- rare or unusual cases may not be seen by trainees, unless called in by the coach to witness them
- advice-seeking potentially provides a significant opportunity for the coach to engage in training, but since the focus of attention is service delivery these opportunities are often left unexploited.

STRENGTHS AND WEAKNESSES OF MODEL 2

When I joined this firm, I went to clinic and was told if I had any problems to get the advice of the Registrar. Well, I was new to the specialty, so at first I hardly knew anything and kept having to ask [the Registrar] what to do. He would tell me, but then he began asking me questions—what I thought about it, what I thought the options were, what I thought would happen if we did this, that or the other to the patient. I hated it at first, because I thought I was giving wrong answers or being made to look stupid for not knowing something obvious. I just wanted him to tell me what to do and then I could do it and get it over with. I realised it was helping me to learn and I did learn from him, but it wasn't easy. In the end, I learned that I could ask him questions and he told me lots of things. In my next job, I think I'll be more confident about asking questions once I've settled in.

Trainee

Normally the trainees will deal with patients themselves if they're happy with it. As soon as there's a problem with the diagnosis or treatment, the trainee can go and have a chat with the Consultant, who will either discuss it or go to see the patient as well. Trainees aren't daunted to come and ask if they're not sure. Some trainees differ a bit on their threshold of when they ask for help and advice. Some like to check every patient through to start with and others may be reticent and not ask often enough. So there's a settling in period when the threshold's being established and it's useful for both sides, Consultant and trainee, to get the feel of whether the trainee's asking too often or not enough.

> *We've not had any particular problem in this regard, but just occasionally it's obvious that a trainee is doing a procedure that they're not quite experienced enough to do or a patient comes back to a later clinic and you wonder whether what the trainee did was the right move at that stage.*
>
> *In a specialty like ours, doctors are working independently in the out-patient setting, so it's difficult for us Consultants to judge how the consultation is going in the next room. If a trainee's having difficulties it usually filters back to us through the nurses. The only way we really observe what's going on in clinic is when the trainee comes along and says 'I don't know what to do about this.' It seems a bit woolly and it would be easier if we had the option of training clinics where the juniors saw a patient and then discussed it immediately.*
>
> Trainers

Model 3 — Service delivery with follow-up training

All doctors engage in service delivery (with or without the filtering of patients), but coach and/or trainee save up interesting cases, issues and questions for discussion during a planned or scheduled break or at the end of clinic.

Advantages are:

- no teaching during service delivery, even when a trainee seeks advice from a coach, so the clinic is very efficient
- the teaching at the end of clinic can be open and relaxed, as no patients are present
- the trainee can, during clinic, construct an agenda of questions for the coach to answer and so be pro-active in shaping the training.

Disadvantages are:

- the training lacks structure and cases discussed at the end may not meet trainee learning needs
- 'cold' teaching at the end of clinic is less effective than 'hot' teaching when trainees seek advice from the coach during service delivery
- the post-clinic discussion is easily dropped or curtailed when the clinic is busy and so runs late, or when the coach or trainee is tired or when either is called away to some other aspect of service delivery.

Model 4 — planned training within service delivery

In this model, training is carefully planned. The trainee:

- contributes to service for those cases or aspects of management where the trainee has known competence and/or has been previously trained
- is given training by the coach on pre-selected topics where competence or experience is lacking.

The topics are pre-selected in accordance with the training plan to form a 'training menu' (see Section 11) for this particular clinic. When either the trainer or the trainee sees a case from the training menu, it serves as a 'trigger' for the two to meet to discuss the topic/case.

> *If a junior came along and said 'Look, I've seen this and this, but I need to get this and that' I'd say 'Fine, we've got several cases today and I can show you this during the first case and that during the third case.' The onus needs to be on them to tell us what they need to see not for us to try and show them every case, which is unrealistic.*
>
> Trainer

The 'training menu' topics should not be whole-case management of a particular disease or condition — this would take too long and be impractical — but a selected part of the management appropriate to the patient, e.g. if a new patient — the history or the relevant investigations; if a follow-up patient — the management options or rehabilitation or discharge.

The decision on the training menu is made just before clinic or in a follow-up session to a Model 3 clinic. The menu may not be adhered to in any rigid way — the particular circumstances (including which patients turn up for clinic) will entail making some changes, usually minor ones. At an early point in the attachment, the menu consists of common and relatively simple cases, so that the trainee can quickly make a contribution to efficient service delivery. This creates space for more complex cases to be added to the menu and time for relevant teaching by the coach. In this way, the clinic becomes efficient and trainee progression is also achieved.

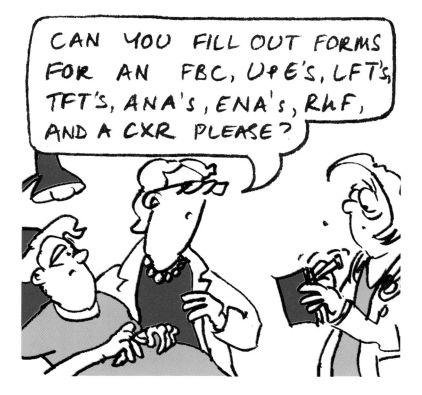

The trainee may see both new and follow-up patients, but the model requires some 'filtering' of patients. This may be done by trainer, trainee or nurses/managers, but requires clear understanding and careful organisation in the detailed arrangements that are made immediately prior to the clinic. With a little practice, and an awareness by all staff of the underlying rationale, this system runs smoothly.

Advantages are:

- the model supports trainee progression, as the filtered cases can change from week to week and increase steadily in difficulty
- the likelihood that trainees will see the range of cases specified in a training plan is increased
- teaching is highly focused, concentrated and less intrusive
- the trainee can seek advice from the coach on menu topics but, based on prior preparation, can then be expected to suggest options for management, including reasons for a preference in the case at hand
- the risk of insufficient time for follow-up discussion is avoided.

Disadvantages are:

- some preparation is needed and also has to be planned into the schedules of trainer and trainee
- the cases that it is hoped will be seen by trainees may not in practice be available at the designated clinic or at a convenient time
- this model requires clear briefing of all clinic staff and meticulous organisation.

Note: much can depend on the clinic's physical layout. If consulting or examination rooms are distant from one another, it may be difficult for trainers and trainees to meet and talk without disrupting service delivery.

Model 5 — the training clinic

Here the trainer reduces the number of patients to be seen and advises those to be seen that the clinic has a teaching aspect to it.

Advantages are:

- trainees receive a considerable amount of tailored training
- informing patients that the clinic is a training clinic encourages open discussion in front of the patient about their condition and allows the trainee to lead the consultation under the direct supervision of the coach.

Disadvantages are:

- the number of patients that can be seen is considerably smaller than with other models
- the trainee has limited responsibility for decision making.

One unusual variant of the training clinic is the combined service and teaching clinic, which has a patient list of particularly difficult or interesting cases, referred by managing hospital doctors or GPs. A team of doctors runs the clinic, and each doctor sees every patient. The consultations are followed by group discussion, in the absence of the patient, and management steps are debated and agreed. The opportunities for trainees to learn are many, and these can be enhanced by the use of skilful questioning and the promotion of a spirit of co-operation and mutual support.

Here is one example of a regional combined clinic which doctors rate highly.

The aims: To pool the knowledge, experience and expertise of specialists in the region, in order to provide the most effective treatment to patients with particularly difficult conditions. To inform the specialist community about 'interesting' cases from which lessons can be learnt. To give second, third, fourth opinions where patients request them.

The context: The clinics take place bi-monthly in two different regional locations. Each clinic is attended by 10 to 20 doctors of all grades from the specialty across the region and other 'interested' individuals are invited to attend.

The procedure: Doctors from across the region may refer patients to the clinic where assistance, advice and/or support with diagnosis and/or treatment is required, or where 'interesting' cases are encountered and they wish to share them with colleagues.

The process: Approximately 10 patients attend each clinic. Each doctor is given a short, anonymised summary of each patient, covering where appropriate, history, examination findings, treatment, test results and reason for referral.

All patients are placed in separate consulting rooms. The rooms are numbered and each doctor visits each patient. The consultation process takes about an hour.

The follow-up session is chaired by a Consultant on a rotating basis, and lasts about an hour. The Chair opens the discussion by selecting one of the trainees (usually) to present their findings, opinions and next step suggestions on the first patient. Using one or two open questions the trainee will be drawn on particular aspects, for example 'What investigations would you advocate?' and 'What therapeutic suggestions would you make?' Consultants and other trainees are invited to comment, suggest or question. As discussion points are raised, contributions are made freely, comparing and contrasting opinions and practice. Following a short discussion, the Chair summarises decisions made and moves the discussion on to the next patient.

113

The follow-up: As a matter of routine particularly interesting cases are noted for feedback on progress at some stage in the future. At the end of each clinic any feedback on previous patients is given.

The benefits of the clinic are that it:

- provides a forum for meeting regularly with trainers, trainees, GPs and other interested individuals to exchange thinking and ideas, and to share problems
- promotes a 'learning community' whereby trainers and trainees learn from and support each other
- demonstrates the diversity of opinions and practices
- encourages trainees to make decisions, offer analyses and learn from more knowledgeable and experienced colleagues
- offers to patients a pool of specialist expertise so ensuring that they receive the most appropriate treatment available.

THE MERITS OF THE COMBINED CLINIC

Firstly one selects interesting cases which are likely to be of educational value. The usual trigger for bringing someone along is when one of us is in the clinic and we're not quite sure what to do, or not quite sure what the diagnosis is. Then each person attending, particularly the trainees, has to decide what they think the diagnosis is for all of them, even though they're only going to be asked about perhaps two or three. Since they don't know which patients they're going to be asked about, they have to grapple with each case, and decide what they think and look very carefully. Having the different possibilities aired—I think that's extremely educational. You get to understand how the more experienced people think, what's going through their minds and why, which is more valuable than being told 'This is a good example of this, there you are'.

Trainer

The style we have—non-aggressive—works best. I think it's stressful enough to have one's possible ignorance displayed in front of one's consultants even when they're being pleasant and relatively jovial. People are more likely to respond appropriately and be prepared to speak up and ask questions in that sort of setting.

Trainer

It's friendly, it's instructive for all levels. The consultants find it useful and the juniors find it useful.

Trainer

> The joint clinics have been really useful; they're real learning. When you first start, you feel a little bit intimidated because you really don't know anything and you're asked to give an opinion. But you get to know everybody. It's a way you really learn. If you say you don't know and you've not seen it before, then you're not made to look stupid, they just move on to the next person and see what they say.
>
> Trainee
>
> They're very good once you get the hang of the real basics which takes a few months. You see how very senior people do it, what the thoughts are that go through their head because they chat about it and you listen in. Everybody enjoys those clinics.
>
> Trainee

The five models in action

Many clinics follow models 1–3 or some mixture of them. Model 1 is often used early in the trainee's experience and then dropped in favour of the preferred or regular model, which the trainer and the clinic staff regard as routine. Model 4 clinics are rare.

From a training point of view, the ideal model is a combination of models 3 and 4, which mirrors the coaching cycle, or model 5.

This may well not always be possible. To achieve sound training, however, any other model used as 'standard' has limitations. Different models are appropriate at different stages in the trainee's development.

> Phases of a coaching cycle
>
> **Planning phase** where coach and trainee decide the aspect of training on which to focus
>
> **Service delivery phase** into which OJT is fused or blended
>
> **Follow-up phase** where coach and trainee review the quality of trainee performance and any training provided and decide what to do in the next training cycle.
>
> Phases of clinic
>
> Before clinic = **planning phase**
>
> Clinic itself = **service delivery phase with OJT**
>
> After clinic = **a follow-up phase**

115

A mixed-model approach

It is difficult, on any one occasion, to provide in clinic a complete coaching cycle as occurs in the combined models 3 and 4. The advantage of the mixed-model approach to organising training in clinic is that all elements of the cycle are indeed covered, but on separate occasions.

The mixed-model ideal achieves many advantages at the cost of the fewest overall disadvantages, but this needs careful organisation and a full explanation to other staff of the reasons for varying the pattern of the clinic. Since nurses and managers are more interested in the predictability and efficiency — using a constant method of getting through clinic in the shortest possible time — it is essential that the trainer explains the organisation of clinic as being both in the interests of such efficiency and in the interests of training the junior doctors.

An example of a mixed-model programme of training in clinic follows.

Early stages

Model 1 (sitting-in) is adopted for one or two clinics, allowing the trainee to see the trainer at work, so that:

- preferred practice is modelled by the coach
- the trainee sees the range of cases, including the less common and those of complex character
- the trainer highlights the most common and relatively simple cases and what the trainee needs to do to prepare to take responsibility for dealing with them.

This is then immediately followed by Model 4 (planned training within service delivery) with a focus on the most common and least complicated cases to achieve a rapid but high level of trainee competence with such cases. This has the effect of increasing trainee confidence in the work of the clinic, enhancing the part the trainee can play in service delivery and preparing the way for progression in training during later clinics.

FOR NEWLY ARRIVED TRAINEES

Don't be put off by anybody who hurries you along in clinic. It is a setting where you are entitled to training. Just explain that once you know how to deal with a case, you'll be quicker with all such cases in future clinics.

Middle stages

The topics on which training focuses are selected from the training plan (written at the beginning of training — see Section 10). It usually needs the trainee to take the initiative in shaping a training menu: the trainee keeps an eye on whether the targets in the plan are being achieved and moulds the training process accordingly.

Either Model 3 (service delivery with follow-up) and/or Model 4 (planned training within service delivery) or a combination are used to allow a focus on those cases necessary to a stepped progression in training. The choice of model may depend on the circumstances and trainee needs. As examples, if trainer or trainee need to leave early, Model 3 becomes inappropriate; but if the trainee needs experience of particular cases to match the training plan, Model 4 is appropriate.

At the end of each week or clinic, the trainee keeps a log of the extent to which the training plan is being achieved. If the plan has been well designed, this takes no more than a few minutes. This activity helps the trainee to plan the menu of topics for the next clinic. Gaps and omissions, once identified, become the basis for making minor changes to the clinic procedure to provide the necessary training opportunity.

An occasional clinic along the lines of Model 3 can be particularly valuable in providing coach and trainee with a convenient opportunity to monitor progress with the training plan and decide on any action needed to ensure its continuing implementation.

Late stages

At this point the trainee's learning is focused on the less common and more complex conditions. As the trainee has now no sense of being a hindrance to service and feels confident that any interruptions of service to seek advice will not be treated as foolish, Model 2 (service-led training) can be used for much of the

117

time. The trainee has a reasonable range of competence, so interruptions of the trainer are likely to be relatively few — thus maximising service delivery — but highly purposeful and rich in training value when they do occur.

All clinics

A 3 minute round-up at the end of every clinic is an inexpensive way in which the coach gives the trainee some 'quality' time to ask questions and discuss problems.

A 3 MINUTE ROUND-UP AFTER CLINIC

It's really helpful. You go through as many cases as you can to your own ability, you ask for help where you need it, but there are other management problems that you might not have time to discuss during the clinic itself, so a few minutes at the end can sort that out. And it's good to have a chance to go through tricky cases. Even where you were sure what it was, it's helpful to be able to talk through a differential diagnosis or even discuss histology or aspects like that. It's not that Consultants aren't willing to talk to you about these things, but it's difficult to pin people down unless it's a real problem. There are things I need answering for myself at the end of clinic, things that I need to look up, but that takes time and one of the bosses can usually answer it easily while it's fresh in your mind if there's this opportunity for a short chat.

Trainee

At any clinic there are questions that trainers and trainees can usefully bear in mind.

Aide-mémoire **for coaches in clinic**

for each case

- is this on the trainee's menu for today?

- If so, what action might I usefully take?

  - pass the patient over to the trainee
  - supervise the trainee managing the patient
  - invite the trainee in to observe my demonstration of sound examination, investigation, diagnosis, management etc.
  - keep notes on desk for discussion in post-clinic follow-up, especially where issues are most easily discussed in the absence of a patient—e.g. defence litigation, compensation, family circumstance, sensitive prognosis, etc.

- Don't forget the 3 minute round-up.

Aide-mémoire for trainees in clinic

- Have I made out my training menu for today?

- Has it been agreed with my coach or is it just my own?

- Which way of organising the clinic is:
  — appropriate to meeting my training needs
  — practicable and convenient to all affected by it?

- Before seeking advice from the coach, have I thought ahead and worked out the options or possible answers so that I can:
  — demonstrate that I have given some thought to the matter before going for advice?
  — check whether I had worked the answer out for myself?
  — understand better why I was mistaken when my answer proves to be off beam?
  — ask the coach a sensible question to improve my understanding and reasoning?

- Remember that you learn more if you allow the coach to approve or correct your thinking than if you simply ask *What do I do with....?* to get his/her advice on what to do

- Remember the 3 minute round-up

ACTION POINTS ON OJT IN CLINIC

TRAINERS

- before or at the beginning of clinic choose a clinic model:
    model 1—sitting in (no service role for trainee)
    model 2—service-led training
    model 3—service delivery with follow-up training
    model 4—planned training within service delivery
    model 5—the training clinic
  and make sure everybody knows which model you have chosen for what reasons

- apply the appropriate clinic model to match the trainee's learning needs and point of progress to the circumstances and pressures prevailing at the time

- always use a 'training menu' to ensure that the trainee gets OJT from some part of the clinic

- give your trainees a copy of the aide-mémoire for trainees in clinic so that they take more responsibility for their learning

- keep nurses and other staff informed as to the purpose of variations in your adopted models for clinic

- make sure staff understand how, in the long term, variation in the clinic model speeds up service

- remember the 3 minute round-up.

13 OJT ON-TAKE

> It is a safe rule to have no teaching without a patient for the text and the best teaching is that taught by the patient himself.
>
> Sir William Osler, Regius Professor of Medicine
> University of Oxford, 1904

THIS SECTION:
- **explains why on-take work is important for OJT**
- **identifies generic skills trainees can develop when on-take**
- **describes how coaching cycles work when on-take**
- **explores two on-take systems for OJT: partial shift and rota**

Emergency on-call is an important, if often very demanding, part of the physician's training. Yet it is rich in opportunities for OJT, many of which remain unexploited. On-call, by its very nature, has a less predictable structure than other settings such as wards or clinics, but the training techniques described in Part Two are no less applicable. Indeed, the lack of formal structure provides a flexibility and variety that makes a valuable contribution to training. On-call is particularly useful for learning some of the generic skills such as resuscitation and common acute emergencies.

> Emergency take I'm sure is where all the trainees get maximum benefit from everyone except the consultant, until the consultant does the post-take ward round—which is why it's very, very important.
>
> Trainer

> Patients admitted as an emergency are usually seen by the most junior member of the firm such as the post registration house officer, seen subsequently and reviewed by the SHO, subsequently possibly the registrar, then the registrar does a ward round—a take ward round—at ten o'clock at night, or whatever—goes through all the patients. There's an awful lot of learning that goes on there because the post-registration house officer has got the case, taken full history, examination, formulated a plan of management and now has to see whether the SHO agrees with that. A lot of training, teaching and learning goes on.
>
> Trainer

Identifying and developing generic skills

The best trainers use this setting to identify and develop a wide range of generic skills.

An important skill which trainees learn is how and when to prioritise patients. This is a form of triage where the sickest and most urgent patients are seen first. Moreover, trainees on-call often need to be in more than one place at a time, learning to delegate appropriate tasks to other staff; good time-management is another skill to be developed.

The effective on-take team relies heavily upon the capacity of the members to work as a team, which means sharing skills and knowledge, and working collaboratively. This builds up loyalty and camaraderie and improves job satisfaction and morale. Trainees need to feel they can ask for supervision and support when they need it. Trainees learn when they do not know, and that calling for advice or help is appropriate when one has reached the limits of one's knowledge or skill.

> Sometimes there are cases I have on call where I feel I need a senior decision, but then it's out of hours and I think 'Do I really have to call them?' On clinical grounds, some-times if you don't have an enormous amount of experience, it is really difficult to say 'This is what it is' and go and tell the patient or the relatives. You always have the feel-ing at the back of your head that the next morning someone will say 'Why didn't you do a CT or call the Consultant?' Sometimes you have to make a decision which cannot be reversed. Once you've taken that path, it's the end of that story, there's a point of no return. It eventually comes down to the fact that I'm scared of making life and death decisions.
>
> Trainee

Opportunities to develop communication skills also arise when on-take. To observe a senior colleague breaking bad news to a patient or relative, counselling the bereaved, liaising with other on-call services or communicating with GPs, adds to the trainees' knowledge-base from which they develop their own communication skills, especially if, after the observation, trainees are encouraged to discuss briefly what happened and what they would do in similar circumstances. Trainers then offer support, supervision and feedback to trainees whilst they, in turn, deal with similar problems.

Clinical problem-solving skills are also developed through OJT during on-take, especially decision-making, investigative and procedural skills. Keeping records of 'interesting cases' or unusual presentations encourages trainees to ask about them or to look things up at a later or more convenient point. A Polaroid camera [with consent] can be very useful for this.

Generic skills that can be developed on-take through OJT

- prioritisation of patients
- delegation
- organisational abilities
- time management
- seeking appropriate and timely advice, support or help
- working as a member of a team
- communication skills

Planning rather than waiting for training opportunities

On-take, like ward rounds and clinics, may be analysed in terms of the three-phase coaching cycle.

Phases of a coaching cycle

- **Planning phase** where coach and trainee decide the aspect of training on which to focus
- **Service delivery** phase into which OJT is fused or blended
- **Follow-up phase** where coach and trainee review the quality of trainee performance and any training provided and decide what to do in the next training cycle.

Phases of on-take

- at the beginning of the take = **planning phase**
- during the take = **service delivery phase with OJT**
- at the end of the take = **follow-up phase.**

123

At the beginning of the take — a planning phase (for both training and service delivery)

A distinctive feature of the planning phase when on-take is the lack of information about the work the team will face during their period of duty. Where referrals are preceded by contact from a GP or via the A&E department, there may be some advance notice, so making it possible to filter admissions to trainees depending on their learning needs and experience.

Teams beginning a period of on-take need a few minutes to set an agenda for OJT appropriate to any opportunities that present themselves. Led by the senior doctor in charge of the take, each trainee identifies those conditions, medical problems or procedures on their current 'training menu' (see Section 11). Using this information the team seeks, wherever possible, to filter or distribute appropriate admissions to individual trainees.

This is achieved only when the senior doctor leading the take identifies (where the team has not worked together before) how he or she intends to run the take, including:

The organisation of the take

- the role each member of the team is to take
- how the work is to be structured and organised
- what trainer and trainee expect of one another
- what opportunities might be available for OJT
- how those opportunities might be exploited.

During the take — a service delivery phase with OJT

It's expected that the registrars run the take and some of them run the take very much from the back, in other words they are there to be called upon but the house officer does all the work and calls the next one up when he's worried and then possibly reviews it. Other registrars like to be in there and getting quite a lot of hands-on.

Trainer

Patients with acute conditions admitted as emergency cases are often seen, at least in the first instance, by the most junior members of the firm. Recognising life-threatening conditions, knowing how and when to act, and how and when to seek support and supervision from others, are essential skills that trainees must learn quickly if they are to manage acute conditions effectively and efficiently. These should be at the top of the menu for new trainees, who quickly repay the training effort since they soon make a more effective contribution to service and thereby find their confidence boosted.

On-the-job training during on-take is provided largely by the doctor who is 'one higher' in the firm or team hierarchy. So in this setting, OJT draws on peers or near-peers to teach and learn from each other: on-take is a setting where most trainees can find opportunities for teaching or learning from other trainees. When they are open with one another about this readiness to share in teaching and learning, such opportunities are more likely to be fully exploited.

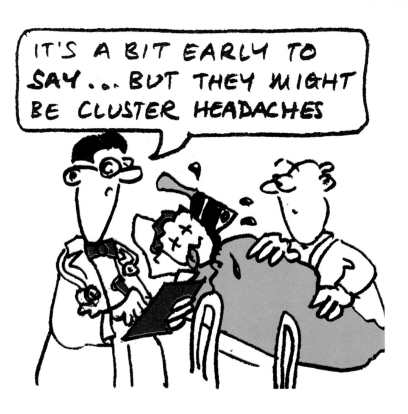

Even when one is very familiar with a procedure, individual patients vary. You can do something for one patient and it all goes like a dream. Then you do exactly the same steps in the same order with another patient and for one reason or another, things don't go like a dream. So if you're a trainee at the bottom of this steep learning curve and you have an awful experience, and then you have another awful experience, you tend to assume it's you and that you're no good and lose confidence, when it may be just bad luck that you've hit two unusually difficult cases.

Trainer

The trainer taught me how to intubate a patient. He took me through it and showed me and I watched it several times. Then he gave me the laryngoscope and said 'You go ahead and do it. The patient is oxygenated, so don't worry, you've got plenty of time.' So I went ahead and if I did it wrong he corrected me. In one case, I couldn't get the tube in so he oxygenated the patient again and put the tube in. He said it wasn't actually difficult, so he took the tube out and gave it to me. He oxygenated the patient again and I had another go. He went through that procedure with me two or three times with different patients that he knew were stable, not too ill. He'd seen the anatomy and knew when it was not easy for me because the patient had no teeth or the neck was very thick and so on. So because there were cases where I could be successful with the procedure, my confidence was really boosted from the very beginning.

Trainee

Opportunities are also affected by the physical circumstances in which the team work. Medical Assessment Units create opportunities for teaching and learning as a result of their single-site admissions, as do hospitals admitting patients to a one-ward location. The lengthy administrative requirements and investigative procedures necessary for each admission means that the on-take team can spend lengthy periods of time in the same location. Trainees who are encouraged to take advantage of the accessibility of more senior colleagues in the on-take team will gain support in their learning.

Regular reviews are a common feature of on-take and an important ingredient of effective OJT. During the review the trainee presents the case to a more senior member of the team, usually at a distance from the patient to ensure privacy. Trainer and trainee then have the opportunity to give and seek explanations (Section 8), to give and get feedback (Section 9) and to ask and answer questions (Sections 6 and 7).

> **During on-take trainers encourage trainees to:**
>
> - scan all service activity for opportunities for OJT
> - present a full and detailed picture of the patient's history, examination findings, assessment and differential diagnoses
> - ask questions and invite opinions about the patient or the condition
> - offer a plan of further investigations
> - formulate possible treatment strategies
> - discuss difficulties/conflicts/complications.

At the end of the take—a follow-up phase for both training and service delivery

This vital follow-up phase often takes the form of a post-take ward round, which offers the opportunity to check diagnoses and management plans. Such teaching is relevant for trainees and often well remembered because it is directly related to patients in whose admission they actively participated. Feedback from the trainer is particularly powerful here, since trainees want to know how well they have performed, and whether their decisions were the right ones. Praise for sound decisions provides the satisfaction associated with professional achievement and corrective advice is taken positively since it can be stored and applied in subsequent on-takes.

Natural tiredness, the pressure of other service commitments or the lack of privacy so easily lead to overlooking trainees' need for feedback on these occasions. Trainers who make the extra effort to provide it when trainees most value it are held in high esteem.

The opportunities for OJT presented by the structure of on-take

> *With a rotation system every team works together very much as a team. They call each other and they say 'Here's something interesting, come and look at this' and they work very much together. And when you get to know how somebody works, it works well. Whereas if you're on-take with somebody that you're not usually on-take with, you don't know how they work so it doesn't work so well. There must be very different ways of running a take and I'm sure some must be more efficient than others for teaching and training.*
>
> Trainer

127

Opportunities presented by the partial shift system

In hospitals operating a partial shift system, on-take teams are, by necessity, made up of individuals who do not work closely together on a continuous basis. One benefit is that each person works with a wide range of trainers and trainees. This has significant potential for OJT; it can facilitate discussion about variations in clinical practice, so making available to trainees a wider range of knowledge and understanding. One constraint is the lack of a shared understanding among trainers of the trainees' interests, strengths and learning needs. Consequently possible planning for OJT, such as the allocation of patients with particular conditions to particular trainees, becomes more difficult. Similar difficulties arise with the follow-up of admissions, since patients are admitted under the care of different teams.

Opportunities presented by the firm or team-based system

Rotation system teams work together on a daily basis, sharing workloads, cases, interests and experiences. The potential for continuity in teaching, building up a secure and comprehensive knowledge-base is greater here than with the changing teams of the partial shift system. However, the continuous hours worked can be longer, leading to exhaustion and reduced learning capacity.

The potential for learning during on-take is considerable. In the hands of a trainer who knows how to exploit the opportunities for OJT, on-take provides the ideal opportunity for combining service with training.

ACTION POINTS ON ON-TAKE

FOR TRAINERS
- at the beginning of every take session, agree training menus with trainees so that admissions can be filtered to them accordingly

- provide specific feedback to trainees on their performance at the end of the on-take or during the post-take ward round.

FOR TRAINEES
- make sure you have a 'training menu' at the beginning of every take, preferably in a short discussion with your trainer, so that you can exploit all the learning opportunities that on-take provides

- identify which generic and clinical skills you wish to improve upon, and alert other team members to these, so that they can be on the look-out for relevant learning opportunities for you

- anticipate all investigative, assessment, diagnostic and management decisions on the patients you admit

- take the initiative: know when and how to ask for help, and don't be afraid to do so—it proves you don't exceed your ability

- be alert to variations in practices and make sure you understand the reasoning behind the differences

- ask for specific feedback from those more senior to you at the end of the on-take session if none is forthcoming.

14 CLINICAL JUDGEMENT, REASONING AND DECISION MAKING

> *Medicine is the most difficult of sciences and the most laborious of arts.*
> Oliver Wendell Holmes, physician, 1871

THIS SECTION:

- **explores the physician's 'cognitive path' in progressing from novice to consultant**
- **examines the concepts of clinical judgement, reasoning and decision making**
- **considers how trainers can help trainees to develop their judgement, reasoning and decision making in OJT**

The postgraduate training of physicians may be characterised as the process by which a novice progresses to becoming a consultant in a specialty or a principal in general practice. Apprenticeship-by-coaching is the partnership between an experienced physician (the coach) and a novice (the trainee) with a view to aiding the latter's progress on the long, slow career to professional maturity. This includes development and change in the way the trainee thinks clinically — a cognitive path.

From the trainee's point of view, training consists of the progressive acquisition of knowledge, skill and understanding. Knowledge is usually easier to acquire than a skill; and a skill is usually easier to acquire than deep understanding. These three concepts, basic to the notion of a cognitive path, overlap in practice. The trainee is regarded as a competent practitioner when a given level of knowledge, skill and understanding has been achieved.

The intellectual path taken by a trainee physician, from registration to the level of the experienced consultant, is under-researched. The process is complicated by the variable level of match between what, on the one hand, the trainer wishes to teach and intends the trainee to learn, and on the other hand, what the trainee wants to learn from the trainer. If trainer and trainee are within the same specialty or sub-specialty, and this is the trainee's intended career route, the match will usually be good and teaching and learning is naturally rewarding to both parties. But where the trainee is not intending to pursue the trainer's specialty, or even sub-specialty, the weaker match may reduce the satisfaction on both sides. Similarly, an SHO preparing for College examinations is often strongly focused on the content of that examination and may well show, during the period of exam preparation, a low level of interest in any teaching and learning in the specialty that is not directly relevant to the exam.

> *Over the next 6 months my orientation is all towards the exam, so I don't really want to learn too much [of this specialty]. I want to learn some, but it's very much a back seat thing. I just want to pass the exam and my efforts are going to be concentrated on that.*
>
> Trainee
>
> *I quite liked the way I was taught. The problem was I was working towards an exam, so I couldn't give it my all. That's a real disadvantage, to work and learn [this specialty] but study for something completely different. Part I exam is on a different plane, it's completely academic and nothing clinical. It's like doing a day job and studying in the evenings for something different, so the day job didn't get all the reading that was probably necessary for it. I had this dual goal, I had to pass an exam and I had to learn [this specialty] at the same time. And after I passed the exam, it didn't make a lot of difference. Everyone said 'Well done' but that was it. You're back to where you were the day before. Nothing changed, even though I had much more interest in learning about [this specialty].*
>
> Trainee

It often requires great sensitivity and skill for the trainer to adapt OJT to meet the specific needs of each individual trainee.

The cognitive path from novice to experienced clinician

This process may be taken to include:

- gaining wider and more extensive experience
- acquiring more relevant knowledge specific to the specialty or domain
- learning to work more efficiently
- making fewer than average errors in assessment, diagnosis or management
- learning to achieve better than average outcomes
- having meta-cognitive skills to think about one's own thinking skills
- thinking creatively within, and questioning, the specialism's conventions
- establishing a reputation that commands the respect of peers.

132

Those who, through a combination of talent, experience and favourable opportunities, meet the above criteria, possess a wisdom that goes beyond the acknowledged competence characteristic of the average consultant.

Clinical judgement, reasoning and decision making of high quality cannot be acquired simply through reading, listening to instruction or observation of a 'master'. Whilst elements of all three are, of course, essential to becoming a competent practitioner, it is the possession of these at the highest level, rather than just more knowledge or greater skill, that mark out the best physicians.

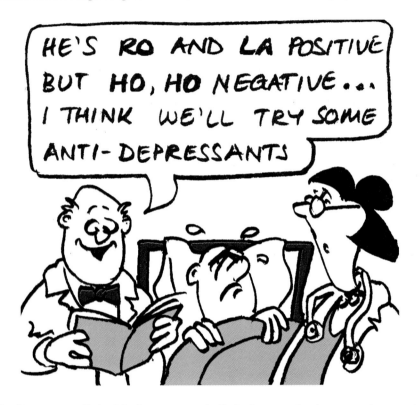

In the literature, clinical judgement and clinical reasoning* are used sometimes as broadly synonymous and sometimes with very different meanings.

* In relation to the associated concept of clinical decision-making, researchers make a distinction between decision analysis and judgement analysis. Decision analysis involves an *a priori* decomposition of the decision process, that is, the decision is separated into its components before the decision is made, such as the clinician's judgement as to the probability and the utility of certain effects of one management option rather than another. Judgement analysis involves an *a posteriori* decomposition that takes place after the decision is reached, such as the weight assigned by the clinician to different pieces of evidence in coming to a diagnostic decision. Most trainers are unfamiliar with this research (see bibliography on p. 149).

133

Clinical judgement is regarded as an important aspect of the end-point to which each trainee is striving and may be taken to mean one or more of the following:

- the ability to make a competent diagnosis and prognosis and to select an appropriate treatment
- the ability, based on extensive and cumulative experience, to make high quality or expert judgement on a regular basis
- the capacity to reason or make judgements on an intuitive, implicit and 'artistic' basis as well as on an analytic, explicit and 'scientific' basis
- the capacity to deploy, in the interests of a particular patient, evidence-based knowledge to complement personal experience of a condition
- the acquisition of high-level meta-cognitive skills, that is, the ability to monitor, reflect upon and change one's way of thinking and reasoning
- the ability to use research on clinical judgement, reasoning and decision making to enhance one's own capacities in relation to each of these.

The associated concept of **clinical reasoning** is used in different senses to refer to a range of cognitive processes.

Sometimes it is used to mean the **hypothetico-deductive** reasoning employed when making a diagnosis, in which the clinician:

- collects data about the patient's condition — signs and symptoms, etc.
- generates one or more (tentative) hypotheses to account for the observed cues
- interprets the data in the light of the hypothesis, which is thereby tested
- evaluates the hypothesis with a view to acceptance, modification or rejection.

Sometimes it is used to mean **pattern recognition**, the **inductive** process by which the clinician recognises, often on an intuitive basis, a pattern in the multiple available data — history, signs and symptoms, X-rays/scans, results of tests and investigations — and thereby reaches a rapid diagnostic conclusion.

> *Everyone who loves clinical medicine and possesses some diagnostic expertise develops a kind of medical sixth sense allowing him or her to discard the irrelevant, to recognise the significant and to be able quickly to collate a constellation of clinical phenomena into a coherent whole.*
>
> Lord Walton, physician, 1993

The preliminary assessment of the diagnostic possibilities stems from the unique qualities of the human mind which is able to take in a very large number of data, to sift their relative significance in an incredibly short time, and to recognise therefrom a pattern... It is skill more closely allied to the skill of a connoisseur examining a picture or an old violin than it is to what we normally think of as science.

Lord Platt, physician, 1972

A tenet of geriatric medicine is that conditions tend to present atypically and a multiple problem is the norm rather than the exception. One needs deductive skills and evidence assessment and collation skills. The temptation is to develop skill with a particular intervention and then to want to apply it just because one knows how to do it. The judgement of when to apply the technology to what extent for which patient is something that some clinicians find hard to acquire. The text-book treatment for a problem isn't always the best, particularly if there are co-existing problems.

Consultant physician

Many patients are elderly and frail with multiple diagnoses. You have to do the best thing by the patient. That requires a great deal of judgement, a certain delicacy and humanity, and the ability to cope with uncertainty, because it isn't necessarily right to treat each condition with the most powerful drug.

Consultant physician

Experienced clinicians probably use both approaches to reasoning in making a clinical judgement, but are bound to use hypothesis-testing when no pattern is recognised. Trainees may not know the pattern or be able to apply the pattern recognition strategy, and so fall back on explicit hypothesis testing and apply a formula-based solution far more frequently than do Consultants.

Research (mainly from North America) suggests, however, that many clinicians are not always as skilful in diagnostic decision making as they (and their patients and peers) might imagine. Since few signs and symptoms are pathognomonic, the clinician has frequently to make a decision from a position of uncertainty by selecting one of several possibilities. It has been shown, to the surprise of researchers, that the use of a simple mathematical formula (linear regression equation) provides a more accurate and reliable diagnosis than experienced clinicians using the same data. This research usefully indicates some of the faulty reasoning that leads to errors in diagnosis, such as:

• assigning significance or undue weight to irrelevant variables
• unduly emphasising data that support a favoured hypothesis

135

- overlooking or discounting evidence that falsifies a favoured hypothesis
- on partial evidence prematurely concluding that a pattern has been recognised
- failing to combine or integrate two or more pieces of evidence
- ordering irrelevant tests and investigations.

All experienced physicians are familiar with these errors in their own clinical experience and encounter them regularly in the reasoning of their trainees.

Happily research also indicates that some clinicians are significantly better than computers in making diagnostic decisions. How these physicians do so is by no means clear, but it seems unlikely that the cognitive processes and strategies they adopt differ from those used by their less gifted peers. Moreover there is no evidence that clinical reasoning is a separable skill, acquired independently of a strong knowledge-base. On the contrary, gains in reasoning ability probably depend on, and are acquired alongside, a growing specialty-specific knowledge-base and its mastery.

It seems reasonable, then, to treat clinical judgement and reasoning as different aspects of a single process or set of processes. *Wise decisions depend on sophisticated judgement arising through sound reasoning and extensive experience grounded on a rich knowledge-base.* Trainees will meet a number of consultant-coaches who regularly make such wise decisions.

Can this be taught? Can it be modelled?

THE VIEWS OF SOME CONSULTANT PHYSICIANS

You can't teach someone to make judgemental decisions.

It's difficult to teach for experience, the business of the art of medicine rather than the science of it. There's an element that is a kind of gut feeling in situations that is very difficult to pass on to a trainee.

Trainers find it difficult to know how to teach reasoning and judgement, especially in any direct or didactic way. Yet it is possible that they can play a greater role than they sometimes allow if the processes involved in this cognitive path are more fully understood. What kinds of knowledge do trainees bring to their training?

Different types of knowledge

Declarative knowledge, or knowledge of facts and events, may be contrasted with **procedural knowledge,** or knowledge of how to do things.

Applicable knowledge tells you what is relevant to a situation; **actionable knowledge** tells you how to implement it in the world of everyday practice.

Trainees acquire text-book knowledge of basic biological and medical sciences; of pathophysiological processes; of conditions and diseases; of drugs and other therapeutic measures and their effects. Much of this knowledge is declarative and applicable knowledge. Trainees have to learn how to transform their declarative and applicable knowledge derived from lectures and books into the procedural and actionable knowledge of clinical practice. This is neither automatic nor easy. It requires work from the trainee; and it can be supported by an effective coach.

The coach can:

- model clinical reasoning and judgement
- 'scaffold' trainee learning by techniques such as questioning
- monitor and provide feedback on the trainee's reasoning and judgement.

The knowledge-base of trainees is too shallow: they need to acquire more declarative and applicable knowledge. Much of this knowledge is acquired through formal training (lectures, presentations, seminars, journal clubs, private study, etc.). This clinical knowledge tends to be stored in packages or schemata — the cognitive structures that contain the general propositions and properties of key concepts.

These schemata are, at the novice stage, only loosely connected and do not constitute actionable or procedural knowledge. Making a diagnosis and a management decision in a real setting is a very different matter: trainees may 'know' in one sense, but cannot, without help or guidance, readily set that knowledge to work in clinical practice. This knowledge is learned on-the-job and through informal training and the help the coach can thereby provide.

'Illness scripts' and the development of clinical reasoning and judgement

Much of our ordinary knowledge is organised in a sequential or narrative form: 'scripts' are fundamental cognitive structures that link facts, events, situations and people (the schemata) in complex sequences to make interconnected wholes.

An illustration of a script.

Take the following three statements.

John goes out for his evening meal.
He chooses the beef.
He leaves a large tip when he pays the bill.

In our culture one 'naturally' reads the three short sentences as part of a sequential story—going to a restaurant—even though this is never explicit and the individual sentences could be part of stories unconnected to a restaurant. The reader 'fills in' much missing detail from an internalised script of 'going to the restaurant' made up of schemata such as 'eating out', 'choosing from a menu', 'rewarding the waiter' which in turn use more basic concepts such as food, menu, tip, bill etc. A Martian unfamiliar with 'going to a restaurant' and lacking its component schemata could perhaps be given a formal lecture about it, but without some practical experience would be very unlikely to manage it as successfully as a native.

Trainees new to a specialty lack some of the specialty-specific concepts; they are strangers to the culture and cannot make sense of all they see and hear. They have to learn new concepts which have to be built into larger schemata related to those already acquired through training and experience; and finally the schemata have to be further developed into the relevant 'illness scripts' — the narratives of the courses of typical illnesses and conditions in the specialty and how they are treated with what consequences. Such illness scripts depend on elements such as:

- the patient's background, history and characteristics
- how the patient presents
- base-knowledge of a text-book type
- diagnostic knowledge of specific signs and symptoms
- results of relevant tests and investigations
- reasoning skills of pattern-recognition and hypothesis-testing

- knowledge of management options and their effects
- knowledge of how to modify the management in the light of the individual patient's circumstances — treating the patient, not the illness or X-ray
- the trade-off between benefits and costs of any therapeutic action.

Illness scripts, built up over many years, are second nature to Consultants. Yet they are not easily taught explicitly: trainees have to acquire them through their clinical practice. Clinical judgement, reasoning and decision making depend on trainee acquisition of these mental representations. Coaching is better than osmosis or didactic teaching alone as a way of teaching illness scripts.

Implications for training

What action might be taken by the coach to help the trainee develop the mental schemata (e.g. illness scripts) and cognitive skills (e.g. hypothesis testing, pattern recognition) that make up the cognitive path of the physician?

In OJT, what the trainer tells trainees or what questions are asked of them tends to be highly fragmented. Consider the schematic illness script set out in the flowchart, which is a simplified model of some of the main components in clinical judgement, following the accepted pattern of the clinician's three basic questions, answers to which provide a comprehensive illness script.

- What is the matter with this patient?
- What can I do for him/her?
- What will be the outcome?

It is the illness script as a whole that the trainee needs to master in order to develop high quality clinical judgement. Yet what the trainee does mostly in OJT touches upon only some of these components — as do the MCQs that lurk in the mind of the examination-conscious SHO. The strength of OJT is that it is learning embedded in the process of making real decisions about real patients. Its weakness is that it is fragmented, and to a degree inevitably so, since service normally focuses on the components of the total illness script that are relevant to clinical action at a specific point.

In consequence the trainee has to collate the illness script from the episodes that arise within service and connect this to what has been acquired through text-book learning, lectures etc. This is no easy task. The scripts are obvious to experts; they are seen darkly through a mist by novices. The fear that many trainees have of being questioned by the trainer or of initiating questions to the trainer is not so much fear of having their ignorance exposed as of appearing to be foolish because what they do know cannot be set with the distinctive rationale of a total illness script that is as yet only partially grasped.

An effective coach helps trainees to learn illness scripts by using three methods of circumventing the obstacle of OJT's endemic fragmentation.

Mastering illness scripts (1): by 'scaffolding' in OJT

The coach has to recognise that those parts of his/her own thinking that are relatively 'tacit' and done intuitively have to be taught quite explicitly to the trainee. For example, in the schematic illness script, experienced physicians often get from **Patient presents** to **Diagnosis made** by the quick and direct route on the right of the table, that is, through instant pattern recognition. The longer left-hand route is used only when the case is difficult or unusual. The trainer needs to take a trainee, who cannot recognise the pattern, through the longer left-hand route in order to learn the diagnostic part of the illness script in an actionable form. The coach needs to be skilful, for example, by asking higher order questions (Section 6) and holistic questioning (Section 7), to 'scaffold' the trainee's learning of this part of the script.

'ILLNESS SCRIPT' COMPONENTS CONTRIBUTING TO CLINICAL JUDGEMENT

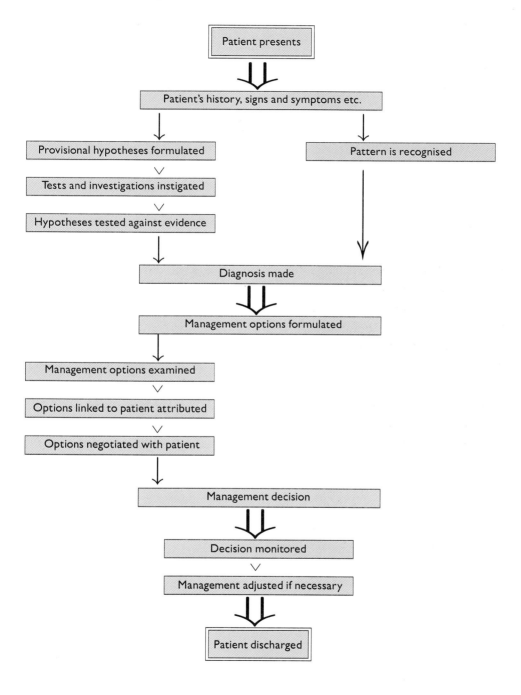

> ## Questions directed to 'filling out' illness scripts
>
> *How did you arrive at that diagnosis? Talk me through your reasoning. Did the patient's age and ethnicity influence your thinking?*
>
> *How do you think I made the diagnosis so quickly? What was the pattern I recognised?*
>
> *How do you think I arrived at my diagnosis? Are you convinced it's the right diagnosis? Are there alternatives we should consider? On what grounds should we decide between the two?*
>
> *You are toying with two diagnostic hypotheses. Is there any difference between them in terms of options for therapeutic management?*
>
> *Now that the tests have clarified the diagnosis, how does it affect our management plan?*
>
> *Why do you think this treatment doesn't seem to be working with this patient? Can you think of other patients with whom it might have been more effective? With hindsight,*

Mastering illness scripts (2): by use of training menu

By using a training menu in clinic or on a ward round, the coach helps the trainee to concentrate and focus learning on just one disease/illness/complaint or a small number of them. On arrival in the specialty or sub-specialty, the trainee is directed to mastering the relatively simple examples of the most common conditions and their management, which rapidly gives the trainee confidence and of course ensures a more effective early contribution to service. Over time, the coach changes the focus progressively to more complex and rarer conditions. Early acquisition by the trainee of whole illness scripts rather than fragments makes teaching and learning the more difficult scripts less onerous.

Intensive focus on a small number of scripts allows the coach:

- to ensure that trainees justify their suggested diagnosis/management (if the suggestion is right, to confirm that both reasoning and conclusion are sound; if wrong, to explore and correct both the suggestion and the reasoning behind it)

- to explore the process of pattern-recognition, or hypothesis-testing, or both
- to show that hypothesis-testing is a way forward if the trainee cannot recognise a pattern
- to encourage the trainee to think out several hypotheses rather than being stuck with the first one they think of — and to give the trainee time to do so
- to persuade the trainee to test the most obvious hypothesis first, and to look for disconfirming as well as supportive evidence
- to get the trainee to check all the hypotheses as fully and systematically as possible to prevent premature closure on a favoured hypothesis
- to help the trainee to learn that ruling out one hypothesis may rule out others too — hypotheses can be nested and tested in logical and economical ways to help the trainee to recognise the possibility of multiple illnesses.

Mastering illness scripts (3): by tracking selected patients

Illness scripts and the associated clinical reasoning are more likely to be acquired by trainees if a range of patients are seen in depth over time. In many specialties this is difficult to achieve, though trainers recognise the importance of doing so.

> Nowadays the pressure is not to bring patients back to clinic for follow-up but to get them back to their GP. Yet it's a very important part of the learning process for juniors to see the patient from the beginning, start the treatment, see how it goes, alter it if necessary and so on. They learn by seeing the same patient again and again. If they don't see the patient again, they don't know if it's worked or not, so in a sense they're not learning through experience at all. To learn by experience requires seeing patients through the whole process. You have to see patients in the natural evolution of the disease, especially if you want to be confident that you're safe to discharge them.
>
> Consultant Physician

The trainee is encouraged to track selected patients from admission to discharge, which of course includes both clinic and ward, whenever this is possible. Among the selected patients there need to be atypical cases.

> *Nine out of ten cases are straightforward, the patients are not severely ill and treat-ment is not very difficult. But there will be a few cases that are much more tricky and require a lot of thought—that's where judgement comes into play. This is one of the things to learn: how to recognise an ordinary case and how to recognise one where things might spin out of control. Some juniors seem to think all they need is run-of-the-mill experience and they've 'done' a disease when they've seen half a dozen simple cases. Actually they need to see a dozen simple cases and a few severe types in order to learn what they can't do as well as what they can do. We have to make sure they get a feel for the whole spectrum.*
>
> Consultant Physician

By these three methods the coach ensures that depth of training is not sacrificed to breadth and progression in the acquisition of clinical judgement is secured.

Education and training: creating a training culture

Novices expect to be trained: they want the knowledge, techniques and skills that mark the competent medical practitioner, and training, both on and off the job, is an appropriate way of obtaining them. Novices' attitudes to their learning and the way they are taught tend to be short-term, specific, instrumental, utilitarian, extrinsic — the demands of the next examination, the next post, the next case, the next day. They are thus sometimes impatient with what their coaches see as the broader education that is necessary to their professional development.

In the later stages of the Specialist Registrar grade, with examinations happily past and most of the core knowledge, techniques and skills of the specialty or sub-specialty in one's grasp, the trainee's outlook inclines more favourably to education rather than training — learning that emphasises the longer-term, the complex, understanding rather than knowledge, the problem or the solution that is intrinsically interesting rather than immediately useful.

A group of Consultants who see themselves as learners and who are committed to the training of their juniors create a culture of training, in which it is evident that learning is highly valued and a natural concomitant to high quality service. When service is seen by the coaches as a source of learning for themselves, it will be so seen by trainees, and the simplistic antithesis between 'training' (i.e. uninterrupted

144

by service) and 'service' (i.e. which excludes training) is defeated. Training can be dry and difficult to apply when it is divorced from practice; service can simply be 'work' when it is disconnected from learning. A learning culture does not necessarily mean more formal teaching or more direct supervision by consultants or a lower service commitment from trainees. It means the environment is one in which opportunities for learning and the importance of learning pervade the work of all, whether the activity be called service, on-the-job training or formal teaching.

The acquisition of clinical judgement by the Specialist Registrar is an important objective in the education of a physician. It is in this area of improving judgement through OJT that the closest professional bond is created between Consultant and trainee. The most outstanding coaches, through their infectious enthusiasm for their work, their commitment to teaching and their willingness to share their expertise, undoubtedly educate as well as train their juniors. They openly continue to learn — from any source. It is with good reason that the later stages of learning in medicine are usually referred to as continuing medical education (CME), which is aided by growing experience and the on-the-job learning that is enhanced by training others.

> One thing that worries me about the notion of 'being trained' is that it sounds like an end-point. I remember the father of my specialty saying that the day he did a clinic and didn't understand something for the first time, he would retire from clinical practice. It's a level of competence you reach after you've been trained, not an end-point. You have to keep on going with your learning. And I'm bound to say that you can learn far more from your juniors than attending meetings that are officially part of your CME. I had superb training and when I was a houseman I was struck by the friendship between the senior surgeon and the senior physician. They used to do a Saturday ward round together and if one had a difficult patient he would take the other to see that patient simply to give another eye on the clinical problem. That struck me as extraordinarily sensible. That's how you learn.
>
> Consultant
>
> For people to learn in medicine, they have to be the sort of people who always want to learn. That's not the same as having the skill to pass an exam, which is more superficial. We need to be taught how to learn, how to educate ourselves all the way through. It's getting people into a learning mode. Catch them early and the rest follows. Getting positive feedback and feeling motivated, then you learn.
>
> Trainee

145

Such a culture plays an important role in transforming training into education. Effective OJT, where service is the medium of training, is the principal support of an educational environment and training culture in which everybody learns.

For a select bibliography on the themes of this Section, see p. 149.

15 CONCLUSION

> *We have outrun an educational system framed in simpler days and for simpler conditions. The pressure comes hard enough upon the teacher but far harder upon the taught, who suffer in a hundred different ways.*
>
> Sir William Osler
> Regius Professor of Physic, Oxford, 1913

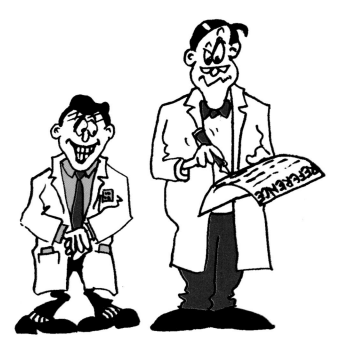

The environment in which physicians are trained is changing. Hospitals are busier and increasingly driven by the need to meet service contracts; the period of training is shorter; and hours of work are restricted. To maintain standards, the quality of postgraduate medical training will need to be improved. To this end physicians will need to strike a new balance between the various approaches to teaching and learning:

- formal and didactic teaching, presentations, seminars, etc.
- journal clubs
- courses
- private study

147

- on-the-job training
- research and audit.

Given the time constraints, improvement must mean better OJT, not just more formal training. Changing from apprenticeship-by-osmosis to apprenticeship-by-coaching poses the greatest challenge. Effective OJT requires a distinctive relationship between coach and trainee, and this has five principal features:

- the coach makes maximal use of the opportunities for teaching that become available during service
- the trainee takes greater initiative in a similar search for, and use of, learning opportunities and is skilful in eliciting teaching from the coach
- the coach is skilled in selecting an appropriate teaching technique (questioning, explaining, demonstrating etc.) in a particular setting (ward, clinic) for a chosen training focus (the training menu of the day) within a progressive sequence of training (the training plan)
- there is regular feedback provided in a variety of forms. The trainee has a strong sense of progression in learning and a record of it
- training is minimally disruptive of service delivery because wherever possible OJT is fusional.

The various forms of OJT are at the centre of postgraduate medical training because they link training to patient care. The close relationship between OJT and service offers the opportunity for the development of, and education in, the most elusive of the physician's skills—reasoning and judgement. The challenge to both consultants and specialist registrars is to make the changes necessary for creating the high quality OJT that can play such a key role in the training of physicians.

> *New ideas build their nests in young men's brains.*
> Oliver Wendell Holmes, physician, 1871

Clinical judgement, reasoning and decision making: a select bibliography

Argyris C, Schön DA. *Theory in practice: increasing professional effectiveness*. San Francisco: Jossey-Bass, 1974.

Arkes HR, Hammond KR eds *Judgement and decision making*. Cambridge: Cambridge University Press, 1986.

Downie J, Elstein A eds *Professional judgement: a reader in clinical decision making*. Cambridge: Cambridge University Press, 1988.

Eddy DM, Clanton CH. The art of diagnosis. *N Engl J Med*, 1982; **306(21)**: 1263–8.

Elstein AS, Shulman LS, Sprafka SA. *Medical problem solving: an analysis of clinical reasoning*. Harvard: Harvard University Press, 1978.

Engelhardt HT, Spicker SS, Towers B, eds *Clinical judgement: a critical appraisal*. Dordrecht: D Reidl Publishing Co, 1979.

Ericsson KA, Smith J, eds *Towards a general theory of expertise*. Cambridge: Cambridge University Press, 1991.

Evans DA, Patel VL, eds *Cognitive science in medicine*. Cambridge, MA: MIT Press, 1989.

Feinstein AR. *Clinical judgement*. New York: Robert E Krieger, 1967.

Gale J, Marsden P. *Medical diagnosis*. Oxford: Oxford University Press, 1983.

Higgs J, Jones M, eds *Clinical reasoning in the health profession*. Oxford: Butterworth/ Heinemann, 1995.

Kassirer JP, Kopelman RI. *Learning clinical reasoning*. Baltimore: Williams & Wilkins, 1991.

Llewelyn H, Hopkins A, eds *Analysing how we reach clinical decisions*. London: Royal College of Physicians of London, 1993.

Macartney FJ. Diagnostic logic. In: Phillips CI, ed. *Logic in medicine*. London: BMJ Publishing Group, 1988.

Schank RC, Abelson RP. *Scripts, plans, goals and understanding*. Hove: Lawrence Erlbaum/ Wiley, 1977.

Schön DA. *The reflective practioner: how professionals think in action*. New York: Basic Books, 1983.

Schön DA. *Educating the reflective practitioner*. San Francisco: Jossey-Bass, 1987.

Spiegelhalter DJ. Formal representations of medical knowledge clinical judgement. In: Phillips CI, ed. *Logic in medicine*. London: BMJ Publishing Group, 1988.

Vieuten CPM van der, Newble DI. How can we test clinical reasoning? *Lancet* 1995; **345**: 1032–4.

149

ACKNOWLEDGEMENTS

The University of Cambridge Training of Doctors in Hospitals Project is sponsored by the Postgraduate Dean, Dr JSG Biggs, and funded by the Anglia Postgraduate Medical and Dental Education Committee.

We acknowledge with gratitude the assistance and advice of the following, who contributed to the ideas, the development of practice, the field-testing and criticism of the emerging text. We are of course entirely responsible for the shortcomings of the work.

Consultant Physicians

Colin Borland, Christopher Byatt, Timothy Cox, Adrian Crisp, Richard Dickinson, Julian Fasler, Susan Forster, Sunit Ghosh, Alex Gimson, Ray Godwin, Steven Gray, Ian Hardy, John Kneeshaw, Raymond Latimer, Jonathan Mackay, Paul Norris, Amo Oduro, Richard Pye, Paul Siklos, John Stark, Jane Sterling, Pamela Todd

Specialist Registrars/Senior Registrars

Emil Cardan, Toddy Daly, John Francis, David Hildick-Smith, Farhani Ismail, Igrar Ismail-Zade, John McIntyre, Nilofer Mahmood, Quentin Milner, Robert Sarkanay, Simon Shields, Michael Simmonds, John Urquhart, Sarah Woodrow

Senior House Officers

Christopher Browning, Amanda Hagley, Susan Halfpenny, Steven Harris, Helen Hobbiger, Melissa Holden, Rebecca Holden, Mathew Hynes, Lucy Mackenzie, Clare Murphy, Clemens Overlack, Robert Paris, Nicholas Swale, Sean Weaver, Angela White

Project Team Members

Joy Anderson, Martin Booth and Howard Bradley

BIOGRAPHY

David H Hargreaves is Professor of Education in the University of Cambridge and a Fellow of Wolfson College. He is a Director of the University of Cambridge Project on the Training of Doctors in Hospitals and the author of numerous books and articles in learned journals on professional and institutional development.

Geoff Southworth is Professor of Education designate in the University of Reading and a co-director of the University of Cambridge Project on the Training of Doctors in Hospitals. He is the author of many books and articles in learned journals on professional and institutional development.

Paula Stanley is a Research Associate in the University of Cambridge School of Education and is a member of the University of Cambridge Project on the Training of Doctors in Hospitals. She has been a Research Officer at Cranfield University School of Management, where she was involved in public and service sector management research. She is the author and co-author of a number of articles and reports arising from these projects.

Simon J Ward is a Member of the Royal College of Physicians (UK) and a Fellow of the Royal College of Surgeons of Edinburgh. He trained at Cambridge and King's College Hospital Medical School, London. He has undertaken postgraduate degrees at the Institute of Child Health, London and Gonville and Caius College, Cambridge. He is associated with the Project on the Training of Doctors in Hospitals.